HEALTH SECRETS

FOR THE

21st CENTURY

Volume Two

Surviving Modern Times

K.W. PETERS

First drafts edited by Sarah Brooks and Will McLellan

ISBN: 978-0-9866158-3-2

Printed and bound in Canada.

Written by Kenneth Walter Peters.

First drafts edited by Will McLellan, and Sarah Brooks.

Author's photo, and cover, by Sarah Brooks.

Book Design by BookDesign.ca.

Dedicated to Sarah Brooks,
for helping me become a better writer.

Contents

PART ONE
ESSENTIAL SUPPLEMENTS

PART TWO
RADIATION AND
XENOESTROGENS

PART THREE
ELECTROMAGNETIC
POLLUTION

INTRODUCTION

"The end of the human race will be that it will eventually die of civilization."

Ralph Waldo Emerson

As you may have noticed, Volume 2 of Health Secrets For The 21st Century is subtitled "Surviving the Modern Age". In this volume I will first look at a few nutrients chronically absent from our lives, and critical for our wellbeing (iodine, magnesium, and vitamin K2), as well as one hormone (melatonin). I believe, in order to remain healthy, we need to use all these compounds, in supplemental form. These elements are essential, and are not provided by our diets in adequate amounts (due to various detrimental aspects of modern life).

Following this I will examine the omnipresent dangers of electromagnetic pollution, radiation, and hormone disrupting chemicals—all under-reported perils, ever more rapidly growing, and compounding.

In the chapter focusing on Dirty Electricity, we discover the theory that much of modern illness can be attributed to the dawn of widespread electrical usage—in which case Emerson's quote may prove to be frighteningly prescient. Now that we have cell phone towers, wireless emissions, high levels of ionizing radiation in the environment, and damaging xenoestrogens migrating into our bodies, his quote seems even more relevant.

THE DISINFORMATION AGE

As mentioned in Volume One of Health Secrets for the 21st Century, and as those who read my blogs (www.nutristart.com) know, I believe there is an active disinformation campaign targeting nutritional supplements, which issues directly from pharmaceutical companies. I would add, there is also collusion with the media in this—either that, or journalism is so listless now, it cannot be bothered to fact-check anymore.

Those with only a basic interest in nutritional supplementation could be forgiven for throwing up their hands and giving up on trying to determine which supplements are good, bad, or worthless—especially given conflicting research, and misleading headlines, concerning such research.

I also mentioned, in Volume One, we have to keep up on our learning, and research, since the information does often change, and sometimes that new information is valid.

In the following chapter, I will give three examples of poor research, given widespread media exposure, which I was able to refute easily (usually with just a look at the actual study, and a basic understanding of nutrition).

Although I am not a doctor common sense, and access to sites like PubMed (in order to view the original studies in question), provided me with enough material to refute these so-called "scientific" studies. As you will see, to call these studies "scientific" is to bring disrepute to the term. The questionable studies to follow are so flawed and one-sided, one could easily believe they were designed to do nothing but destroy the reputation of certain nutritional supplements.

Have a look at the three examples (one extensive, and two brief) to follow, which you may have read about in the media, and which may have caused some doubt in your mind. After setting your mind at ease regarding the value of nutritional supplements, we will explore the use of nutrition, and alternative technologies, to cope with the many dangers inherent in modern living.

DISINFORMATION

VITAMIN D UNDER ATTACK

"Vitamin D supplements don't help boost bone density in healthy adults." This headline, from a few years ago, refers to a study published in The Lancet Medical Journal (from the University of Auckland's Department of Medicine, NZ). The headline was splattered all over the internet for days afterwards (not to mention countless newspapers), with little or no critical response (outside of D-specific websites, like The Vitamin D Council).

The study was actually a review of 23 other studies, looking at 4,082 patients (most of them women) taking supplemental vitamin D for an average of two years. The overview found little difference in bone density (measured at key points in the skeleton—the hip, the forearm, or the lumbar spine).

"The negative findings of our analysis contrast with the widely held perception that vitamin D works directly on bone cells to promote mineralization," the scientists wrote. "This perception is probably incorrect." (1)

FLAWS IN THE NEW ZEALAND BONE DENSITY STUDY

Now, let's have a look at the main flaws in this very unscientific attack on vitamin D.

First, we are looking at a pooling of various studies, conducted all over Europe and the U.S.—so we have no indication of how many people lived in areas where they received sufficient sunshine for D production. Nor do we have any idea what amounts of vitamin D their diets might have provided.

All these people may have already been deficient in vitamin D, which is likely since it has recently been shown vitamin D deficiency is rampant, even in countries with lots of sunshine throughout the year—such as India (80% deficient), and Oman (87% deficient). As the subjects in the studies reviewed lived mostly in the temperate zone, the odds are a good many of these people were already very low in vitamin D.

In almost half of the studies reviewed, the amount of vitamin D given as a supplement was insufficient to make a difference—especially if the subjects were already D-deficient.

According to the New Zealand review, "In ten studies, individuals were given vitamin D doses less than 800 IU per day". Compare this to the 10,000 IU of vitamin D your body can make from 30 minutes of direct sunlight (with proper sunbathing, at the proper time of day, and year), if you are deficient.

COUNTERSTUDY

This study also ignores one from the previous year, which found that people 65 and older, who took 800 to 2,000 units of the vitamin daily, had a 30% lower risk of hip fractures. In that study, they found taking less than 800 IU of vitamin D per day (with or without calcium), had no effect on bone-fracture risk, when compared with taking a placebo, or a calcium supplement alone.

However, taking 800 IU or more, on a daily basis, decreased the risk of hip fracture by 30%, and the risk of other bone fractures by 14%. "A 30% reduction in hip fracture with an inexpensive and safe intervention such as vitamin D has enormous public health implications," said the lead author Dr. Heike Bischoff-Ferrari, director of the Center on Aging and Mobility at the University of Zurich, in Switzerland. (2)

A comment from the doctor who wrote an editorial accompanying this vitamin D study, really hits the nail on the head—and could as easily be applied to the flawed study from New Zealand: "All of the problems with previous studies come from a very modest dose of vitamin D. If you don't give [study participants] enough of the vitamin D, then you won't see an effect."

BLOOD LEVELS OF VITAMIN D

The next flaw in the New Zealand study (aside from nearly half the subjects receiving insufficient vitamin D), is found in this statement: "Mean baseline serum 25-hydroxyvitamin D concentration was less than 50nmol/L in eight studies."

Experts on supplementing with vitamin D, such as The Vitamin D Council (www.vitamindcouncil.org), and Life Extension Foundation (www.lef.org), believe people should maintain a vitamin D blood level of at least 50ng/ml.

Now, notice the New Zealand study in question here uses a different measurement from that of the groups I have listed. However, once converted (from nmol/L, to ng/ml) their baseline concentration of 50nmol/L, is equivalent to 20ng/ml (in the clinical terminology used by The Vitamin D Council, and the Life Extension Foundation).

This reveals the blood levels of vitamin D in the subjects from the New Zealand study, were clearly too low to be of value in preventing any ailments related to vitamin D deficiency.

As another study confirms, 800 IU of vitamin D will not bring blood levels up to the amount necessary for good health, and good bone density: "Administration of 800 IU of vitamin D3 during 45 days was more effective than D2 in increasing 25OHD, but both failed to achieve adequate levels of 25OHD (= 30ng/ml)." (3)

STUDY ALSO USED VITAMIN D2

Finally, this flawed study looked for existing trials "assessing the effects of vitamin D3 or D2, (but not vitamin D metabolites) on bone mineral density". It is now known vitamin D2 is inactive, relatively ineffective as a D supplement, and, in fact, reduces blood levels of D3.

A study reported in the American Journal of Clinical Nutrition—certainly peers of those who produced the New Zealand study—came to this conclusion: "However, the inefficiency of vitamin D2 compared with vitamin D3... at increasing 25(OH)D is now well documented, and no successful clinical trials to date have shown that vitamin D2 prevents fractures." (4)

So, we also do not know what percentage of the studies examined were analyzing blood levels of vitamin D2, an ineffective form of vitamin D.

Given the above material from the AJCN, I have to ask, *do these scientists not compare their own research to that of their peers, before publishing,* or, was this a deliberate hack job, designed to do nothing but discourage people from using vitamin D as a supplement?

Of the vast number of headlines that circulated the world, devaluing vitamin D and its impact on bone density, I could find only one countered by a moderating view (outside of The Vitamin D Council website).

DELIBERATE DISINFORMATION?

The poor quality science used in this flawed study is, for me, enough to consider it a deliberate act of disinformation by a group with a vested interest in maintaining illness in the general population. A cursory check of the study indicates it was sponsored by the New Zealand government, in order to "support the health of its citizens". If that is true, they are getting poor value for their money—or their organization has been co-opted by outside interests (namely those selling drugs for osteoporosis).

REFUTING THE PROSTATE CANCER AND VITAMIN E STUDY

Now on to our second example. A study released in 2011 convinced many people (including the local branch of the Prostate

Society) that taking vitamin E could contribute to developing prostate cancer. This study—along with a bold headline—appeared in most newspapers (and throughout the internet), with no follow up, or opposing opinions.

According to this study, men who took 400 IU of vitamin E daily (during the 7 years they were monitored), were 17% more likely to develop prostate cancer than men who did not take the supplement.

Titled "Prostate cancer risk linked to vitamin E", this study was easy to refute by simply finding the original study on PubMed (Ann N Y Acad Sci. 2004 Dec; 1031:234-41: "Selenium and vitamin E cancer prevention trial." Klein EA).

Here it was revealed the study used synthetic, petroleum-derived vitamin E (racemic alpha-tocopheryl). No one familiar with how to use vitamins would ever recommend the use of synthetic vitamin E. This form of vitamin E is not only ineffective, but may also block vitamin E receptors in the body from up-taking natural vitamin E.

COUNTER-STUDY

As mentioned in Volume One of Health Secrets, if I see a study that swings one way, I can most likely find one that states just the opposite. For example, on PubMed I also found another study (involving over 35,000 men followed for a decade) showing a distinct protective advantage (against advanced prostate cancer) from taking 400 IU of natural vitamin E daily. (5)

STUDY ON WOMEN AND MULTIVITAMINS

Another alarming headline (2011), based on the Iowa Women's Health Study, was titled "Women who use multivitamins run risk of earlier death". This study, which looked at the health of more than 38,000 older women, found women who regularly took multivitamins were 2.4% more likely to die than those who did not (over the 19 years of the study).

First off, the average age was 61, so perhaps the study should have been titled, "Senior Women who use multivitamins run risk of earlier death".

Secondly, the mortality risk was highest among those who took iron in their multivitamin. Any senior woman, purchasing a multivitamin in any reputable vitamin store, would likely be sold one containing no iron. It has been well established, in the field of nutrition, that iron can be dangerous for postmenopausal women, since excess iron has been linked to heart disease.

Finally, the increase in death rate was 2.4%, which verges on statistically insignificant, and hardly worth alarmist headlines. The study also did not take into account the fact many people only begin taking vitamins when they develop health issues. Clearly, if you are elderly, the odds indicate you are more likely to have a pre-existing serious ailment than those who are younger.

Both the vitamin E/prostate cancer study, and the multivitamins/women study, emerged on the same day. Ironically, on the page opposite these articles, in my local newspaper, were two quarter-page ads for drug companies (one for Pfizer, and one for Nicotine replacement therapy with antidepressant options). Perhaps this is why they never printed my letter to the editor explaining the flaws in these studies: they know which side their bread is buttered on.

DO YOUR OWN RESEARCH

I recommend the PubMed website (www.pubmed.com) for those who want to find answers when studies like these, creating confusion and doubt, show up. A free site, "PubMed comprises more than 24 million citations for biomedical literature from MEDLINE, life science journals, and online books", and includes studies from all over the world.

When you see a study quoted (and you question its claims), enter the title into the Pubmed search engine, and have a look at the actual study being referenced. Find out what forms of nutrients were used (i.e. natural, or synthetic). Was the amount sufficient, or too much? What is the nature of the study: was it doubleblind, placebo controlled, or is it a review of other studies? Does the study ignore some key issues related to the subject, such as giving high amounts of one nutrient that requires a co-factor, which was not included?

Vitamin A studies are a classic example of this type of flawed study. Vitamin A in isolation breaks down bone, so studies that use it alone conclude it contributes to osteoporosis. However, vitamin A relies on the presence of adequate vitamin D, which uses the broken down bone material to reconstruct new bone (along with help from vitamin K2).

Taking responsibility for our own health requires we educate ourselves and stay on top of new material in the field, while keeping alert for flawed, misleading, data. It may be a job, but there is no more important job, since all of the joys of life are predicated on being healthy enough to enjoy them.

DEATH BY MEDICINE

"One of the first duties of the physician is to educate the masses not to take medicines."

Sir William Osler M.D.
("The Father of Modern Medicine"; 1849-1919)

MEDICINE AS RELIGION

In 1979, Dr. Robert Mendelsohn published "Confessions of a Medical Heretic", an accurate criticism of the medical profession that is even more valid today. His early warning about our unthinking acceptance of medical advice, prescriptions, and procedures, is confirmed by a modern study titled *Death by Medicine*.

Dr. Mendelsohn firmly believed most drugs are dangerous, and unnecessary, as are most operations. Even just being in the hospital—with its germs, poor diet, emotional stresses, and isolation of the patient from family and friends—is not conducive to healing.

As a "heretic" (one who opposes established doctrines), Dr. Mendelsohn's criticisms of what he called the "Church of Modern Medicine", included these three principles:

- Every drug stresses and hurts your body in some way.

- A healthy society is characterized by strong, positive family relationships, and subsequent minimal need for doctors.

- Doctors are not trained to address the core of any problem, but merely to suppress symptoms.

Dr. Mendelsohn's greatest observation, however, was to point out that Modern Medicine was the new religion. He believed even those who think themselves too rational for religious beliefs, were, in fact, still deferring to unquestioned principles, in the same way religion asks us to.

His analogies of how the religious components related to modern medicine are astute. For example, physicians=priests; research=prayer; medical jargon=sacred language; patient and family histories= confessions; drugs=communion wafers; hospitals=churches; operating rooms=tabernacles; operations=ritual mutilations; non-drug healers=infidels; death=God.

Thus, the doctor/priest is the intermediate step between us, and death/God. He also points out that "Modern Medicine is an idolatrous religion, for what it holds sacred are not living things but mechanical processes". This is evident from the bedside manner of the average doctor—whatever compassion and human touch is to be found in a hospital, usually comes from the "nuns"/nurses.

For a fascinatingly detailed look at the concept of operations being the equivalent of ritual mutilations, see "Altars and Icons— The Surgical Suite as a Sacred Ritual", by Dr. Shawn Tassone (www. drshawntassone.com). And, should you think this to be an absurd concept, consider the study on placebo knee surgery: "Patients with osteoarthritis of the knee who underwent placebo arthroscopic surgery were just as likely to report pain relief as those who received the real procedure." (Department of Veterans Affairs (VA) and Baylor College of Medicine study published in the July 11 New England Journal of Medicine.)

Nowhere is that unquestioning belief in the religion of Modern Medicine more obvious than within the issue of vaccination. For those who belong to this church, questioning the validity of vaccination is like being a Christian, and questioning the existence of Jesus. Otherwise intelligent people are aghast when someone even so much as questions the validity of vaccination—it is akin to heresy.

The stranglehold pharmaceutical companies have on the media is illustrated clearly when the subject of vaccination arises. A recent issue of Maclean's Magazine headlined the subject and—forgoing anything like journalistic objectivity—the article unquestioningly endorsed all vaccines, labeled those who question it as "anti-vaxx-ers", and dismissed them as idiots. There was a time when journalism at least tried to appear it was giving both sides of a story. After all, as you will see, it does not take much research to discover you cannot always trust pharmaceutical companies.

(On the subject of vaccination, I recommend two blogs of mine, available on the Nutristart website, titled, "Protecting Children from Vaccine Injury". This material also applies to adults, and illustrates how taking vitamin C, and/or liposomal glutathione, before and after being vaccinated, can protect one from the potential damage caused by some vaccines. Essentially, if one is in good health using vitamin C will suffice, but if in poor health liposomal glutathione is also required. And never use acetaminophen (Tylenol) following vaccination, as it shuts down glutathione production.)

DEATH BY MEDICINE

In 2004, Life Extension (www.lef.org) detailed a study produced by Gary Null, Carolyn Dean M.D., and three others (including two other M.D.s), titled "Death by Medicine". These professionals ana-lyzed all medical literature concerning injuries, and deaths, occur-ring within the American medical system.

The study was commissioned by the Nutrition Institute of America—a non-profit organization, motivated by the assaults on natural medicine issuing from pharmaceutical companies. The phar-maceutical industry was (and is) running disinformation campaigns in the media, and aggressively lobbying to change laws, in order to deprive citizens of dietary supplements. What their study discovered was shocking to some, but no surprise to many others.

Using only published, peer-reviewed, scientific studies, these researchers added up all deaths caused by adverse drug reactions, medical error, unnecessary procedures, hospital-induced infections, and other related factors. They discovered that total deaths (in the U.S.) caused by conventional medicine was approximately 784,000 per year. This number is greater than the deaths caused by either heart disease or cancer (in 2001, U.S. statistics indicated 699,967 deaths from heart disease, and 553,251 from cancer).

Their conclusion was, "It is now evident that the American medical system is the leading cause of death and injury in the US". (Google-search "Death by Medicine" to find the original article.) Here in Canada, we host the same medical system, only with perhaps fewer unnecessary procedures, since there is less profit motivation in socialized medicine.

CANCER AND HEART DISEASE

My first thought, after reading the aforementioned report, was realizing we also count on the medical profession to help protect us from the two leading causes of death by disease: cancer, and heart disease. However, they do not do a very good job of that, either. Consider that drugs prescribed for lowering cholesterol (in an attempt to ward off heart disease), also rob the body of COQ10, which is required to keep the heart beating regularly. Here the medical approach only leads to heart disease by a different avenue.

Furthermore, we find that, usually within 5 years of a coronary bypass, most of those who previously underwent this procedure have clogged arteries once again. This problem reoccurs because no dietary or lifestyle changes are incorporated into post-bypass regimens. So clearly, there is limited value to the conventional medical approach to heart disease.

As far as conventional cancer treatment, 20 years ago it was believed a man would die of old age before prostate cancer would kill him. Now, since they commonly screen, diagnose, and biopsy men, and treat patients with chemo and radiation, prostate cancer has become a leading cause of death. I think the treatment is killing as many (or more) men than the actual cancer.

I firmly believe the conventional cancer treatments of chemotherapy and radiation do more harm than good, offering a horrible reduction in quality of life, in exchange for a slight increase in quantity of life. That increase in life span is proving to be very slight indeed.

A study published in the Australian journal, Clinical Oncology, was a meta-analysis designed to assess the real benefits of chemotherapy, in treatment of adults with the most common types of cancer. The authors concluded, "...in lung cancer, the median survival has increased by only 2 months and an overall survival benefit of less than 5 percent has been achieved in the adjuvant treatment of breast, colon, and head and neck cancers".

Ultimately, they found the contribution of chemotherapy to 5-year survival, in adults, was 2.3% in Australia, and 2.1% in the USA. (Morgan G, Ward R, Barton M. "The contribution of cytotoxic chemotherapy to 5-year survival in adult malignancies." Clin Oncol (R Coll Radiol). 2004; 16(8):549-60.)

Dr. John Bailer is a respected physician, and a recipient (1990) of the prestigious MacArthur Fellowship (also known as the "Genius Grant"), who spent 20 years working for the National Cancer Institute (including time as editor of its journal). While speaking at the Annual Meeting of the American Association for the Advancement of Science, in May 1985, Dr. Bailer had this to say: "My overall assessment is that the national cancer program must be judged a qualified failure... A change at the National Cancer Institute of the kind I am describing... would mean a massive disruption in ideas, in momentum, in the research community, and in the businesses that support that research community."

So, given the ineffectiveness of the modern medical approach to these diseases, I feel we can put a good number of deaths from heart disease and cancer, into the medical profession's lap as well. And let us not forget the vast amounts of money alloted to the medical professions to research cures for these ailments—almost all of which simply goes to drug research.

NOTHING CHANGES

In 2010, some 7 years after the original Death By Medicine study came out, researchers published a new analysis in the New England Journal of Medicine (Nov. 25/10). That analysis found that the medical profession had not changed to any significant degree. The U.S. medical system was still working towards maintaining its status as the leading cause of death and injury in America. Like the previous study, the authors took their data from the heart of the beast—from medical and scientific journals, and from reports by the Institutes of Medicine. Let's look at some of their findings.

- 18% of patients were harmed by medical care.
- 63% of those injuries were preventable.
- 3% suffered permanent injury.
- 8% experienced life-threatening issues.
- 1 in 9 patients developed a hospital acquired infection.
- Antibiotic overuse created infections super resistant to treatment, worsening the picture for years to come.

Add this, from another source: "Hospital acquired infections killed 48,000 patients in 2006 alone, increasing American healthcare costs by $8.1 billion." (Archives of Internal Medicine, 2011)

LEGAL DRUG DANGERS

Approximately 70% of Americans take prescription drugs—around 3.68 billion prescriptions being filled in the U.S. in 2009, averaging nearly 12 prescriptions for every American citizen.

Facing these jaw-dropping statistics, it comes as no real surprise that the majority of deaths caused by the medical industry, issue from the domain of prescription drugs. Some deaths are due to abuse by patients, some due to mistaken use, and some from doctor error. Too many deaths occur from adverse reactions to correct prescriptions, and far too many from drugs that never should have been on the market in the first place.

Among teens, and young adults, in the years between 2000 and 2008, drug-induced deaths more than doubled. During the same time period, among people aged 50 to 69, death from drugs more than tripled. And these were not deaths from street drugs—though among the younger people many of the deaths did occur from abusing prescription drugs like OxyContin, Vicodin, Xanax and Soma. Overdoses from those drugs now cause more deaths than heroin and cocaine combined.

Adverse reactions to pharmaceutical drugs lead to death, or injuries—resulting in 1 out of 5 hospital admissions—and costs the U.S. more than $136 billion per year.

A study released by the Journal of General Internal Medicine (2010), reviewed records from the year 1976 until 2006. What they found was appalling. Nearly 250,000 deaths occurred due to medication errors in a hospital setting. The errors included drug overdose, prescribing the wrong drug, accidentally giving the patient the wrong drug, or medication accidents during medical procedures or surgery.

In 2011, the Los Angeles Times analyzed data from the U.S. Centers for Disease Control and Prevention, on the death statistics from 2009. They found that, while 36,284 people died from traffic accidents that year, 37,485 people died from prescription drugs. For the first time in modern history, it was determined more people died from prescription drug usage, than from motor vehicle accidents.

Prescription drugs (when taken as prescribed in hospitals) are the fourth leading cause of death in Canada (after cancer, heart disease, and strokes), causing about 10,000 deaths a year in this country. Another 10,000 deaths a year in Canada, which occur outside hospitals, are believed to be caused by adverse reactions to prescribed drugs, errors in dosage recommendations, and/or being prescribed an incorrect drug. In Canadian hospitals, one out of four admissions is related to prescription drugs.

Seniors, as a group, are at higher risk of medication error, and more likely to be harmed by such errors. Unfortunately, adverse drug reactions are common in the elderly, especially after being hospitalized. The most common errors are improper doses, and omission (failure to prescribe a drug in a timely manner, or failure to administer a dose before the next dose is due). Even worse, these errors are compounded, due to the likelihood of the elderly to be taking multiple medications (Journal of Gerontology, 2006).

This medical tendency to put patients on multiple prescriptions is the root cause of the excess of adverse responses. One drug leads to side effects, which are then treated with a different drug—and so on. However, no one is studying how these drugs may counteract each other, or what kind of reactions occur when they are combined.

DO DRUGS EVEN WORK?

In 2006, researchers looked at original clinical cancer research published in five top oncology journals, and three top general medical journals (including the New England Journal of Medicine, the Journal of the American Medical Association, Lancet, and the Journal of the National Cancer Institute).

What they found was further evidence you should not trust medical advice from medical professionals. Study results were published (June 2006) in the journal "Cancer", and revealed undisclosed conflicts of interest. Even worse, these conflicts of interest caused researchers to skew study results in the direction desired by those paying for the research.

There is no doubt that drug companies prefer to fund studies resulting in a positive review of a new drug, since the pharmaceutical industry is first and foremost, a business. Of course, many other industries do the same thing: new studies hitting the news, which tout the benefits of coffee, or sugar, or red wine, are usually funded by the industries selling those products.

CONFLICT AFFECTS OUTCOME

The dominant form of conflict of interest, found in 17% of the research, was industry funding of the study. In a further 12% of the reviewed research, at least one of the research authors was employed by the industry, in either the manufacturing or marketing branches of pharmaceutical companies. Those studies where researchers had a conflict of interest were much more likely to show positive findings.

"Given the frequency we observed for conflicts of interest and the fact that conflicts were associated with study outcomes, I would suggest that merely disclosing conflicts is probably not enough," said study author Dr. Reshma Jagsi, an assistant professor of radiation oncology at the University of Michigan Medical School. "It's becoming increasingly clear that we need to look more at how we can disentangle cancer research from industry ties."

"In light of these findings, we as a society may wish to rethink how we want our research efforts to be funded and directed," Jagsi said. "It has been very hard to secure research funding, especially in recent years, so it's been only natural for researchers to turn to industry. If we wish to minimize the potential for bias, we need to increase other sources of support. Medical research is ultimately a common endeavor that benefits all of society, so it seems only appropriate that we should be funding it through general revenues rather than expecting the market to provide."

Other research indicates many of the studies are often wrong anyways. Medical researcher John Ioannidis, of Tufts University (Medford, Mass.), analyzed years of medical studies. He found many of them are flawed by poor design, bad math, and data analysis that served the desired outcome.

According to Marcia Angell, MD, "...conflicts of interest and biases exist in virtually every field of medicine, particularly those that rely heavily on drugs or devices". She put forth a devastating critique of current medical research in an article titled, "Drug companies and doctors: A story of corruption", published by The New York Review of Books (Jan 2009). There she stated, "…it is simply no longer possible to believe much of the clinical research that is published, or to rely on the judgment of trusted physicians or authoritative medical guidelines. I take no pleasure in this conclusion, which I reached slowly and reluctantly over my two decades as an editor of The New England Journal of Medicine".

Thus, we see researchers designing industry-funded studies in a way that is more likely to produce favorable results, and we find they are much more likely to publish positive outcomes than negative ones.

STATIN DRUGS

The dubious value of prescribed medications can be illustrated by examining a drug almost every doctor would be willing to put you on—cholesterol-lowering drugs, known as statins. These include Lipitor, Crestor, and Zocor, and are the most widely prescribed medications in the world.

Statins act by blocking the enzyme in your liver responsible for making cholesterol. Unfortunately, it turns out that we need cholesterol for a variety of functions, including repairing oxidative damage, supporting brain health, and producing sex hormones. Only 30% of our cholesterol comes from diet, alone, the rest is made internally, which indicates it serves some essential functions.

I am not alone in the belief cholesterol does not cause heart disease. It is only when good cholesterol goes bad that we have a problem, and there are many natural ways around this problem, without shutting down the body's cholesterol production.

There are now nearly 900 studies linking statin drugs to a wide range of adverse effects. Reported side effects include anemia, acidosis, cataracts, immune suppression, liver dysfunction, muscle problems, pancreas dysfunction, polyneuropathy (nerve damage in the hands and feet), rhabdomyolysis (a serious degenerative muscle tissue condition), sexual dysfunction, and tendon problems. There is also some evidence that taking statins may increase one's risk for Lou Gehrig's disease, diabetes, and even cancer.

The most well known adverse side effects of statin drugs is muscle tissue degeneration. This occurs because statins rob the body of Co-enzyme Q10. COQ10 is required by mitochondria to produce cellular energy, and works to keep the heart beating regularly. So, by creating a deficiency in an essential nutrient (found in every cell of the body), these drugs lead to other health issues, including muscle weakness, chronic fatigue syndrome, fibromyalgia, and other potential heart problems.

BRAIN PROBLEMS

In 2001, research started to show the importance of cholesterol in the formation of memories. Studies determined some memory loss could be attributed to a lack of good cholesterol in the body. Soon, reports of cognitive problems, and memory loss—associated with statin drugs—started to become common.

We now know the brain requires cholesterol in order for memory formation to function normally, and some people (not just those taking statins) can be lacking in cholesterol. This is one reason coconut oil is used to naturally treat memory loss and Alzheimer's disease. Coconut oil is a naturally saturated fat (unlike hydrogenated fat, which can lead to heart disease), and will raise cholesterol levels in a healthful way.

Dr. Duane Graveline is a medical doctor (and former astronaut), whose health was seriously damaged by statin drugs. As a result, he came out of retirement to investigate statins, which he has been studying for over a decade now. One thing he discovered was, "When a statin is used, it blocks the mevalonate pathway to get at cholesterol inhibition... But in so doing, it blocks CoQ10, 'dolichols', as well as other major biochemicals...".

Dolichols are the major lipid (fatty) component (14% by mass) of human substantia nigra. The substantia nigra is a brain structure, located in the midbrain, which plays an important role in addiction, movement, and reward. Dolichols influence all the hormones involved in mental states (including emotions and moods), and without sufficient dolichol the entire process of neuro-hormone production will be negatively altered.

According to Dr. Graveline, there are thousands of reports of aggressiveness, depression, homicidal impulses, hostility, increased sensitivity, paranoia, and suicide, linked to statin drug use.

And it gets worse: consider someone prescribed a statin drug, who might later become depressed, or start having suicidal thoughts. They tell this to their doctor, and, instead of being taken off the drug, they are prescribed an antidepressant to take *with* the statin. Now we have compounded the problem—a problem that may not have existed at all before the patient was prescribed the statin drug.

Since the SSRI class of anti-depressant drugs (like Prozac) come with a warning that they can double the risk of suicide, stacking something like this on top of a statin drug (which is already is causing neurological break down), verges on criminal.

PHARMACEUTICAL CRIMINALS

Speaking of criminals, the prescription drug industry is exclusively based on financial interests—not what works for your good health. This is clear since serious side effects are routinely ignored (or hidden), and ineffective and/or harmful products continue to be marketed. Let's look at a few examples.

Vioxx was pulled from the market in 2004, as a response to work done by David Graham, associate director of science for the U.S. Food and Drug Administration's Office of Drug Safety. In a study he led (published in The Lancet Medical Journal), it was determined that taking Vioxx increased risk of coronary heart disease by 34%, compared with other anti-inflammatory drugs. Dr. Graham estimated that during the 5 years that Vioxx was sold in the U.S., it caused between 88,000 and 140,000 excess cases of serious heart disease, and about 44% of those cases would have resulted in death.

He also said his supervisors at the FDA attempted to discourage him from presenting these findings saying, "They tried to block it from being published". This is only one example of the problem with governmental regulatory bodies: they are more protective of the financial interests of pharmaceutical companies, than they are of the health of their own populations. (The situation is much the same in Canada, with our version of the FDA, *Health Canada.*)

Another example of criminal behavior among drug companies can be found in an antitrust class action brought against the pharmaceutical giant, Merck. The lawsuit claimed Merck had known for at least a decade that its mumps vaccine was "far less effective" than it told the FDA. As well, Merck falsified test results, and sold millions of doses of its mumps vaccine of "questionable efficacy", while at the same time monopolizing the market. Two ex-employees of Merck (virologists) claimed they "witnessed firsthand the improper testing and data falsification in which Merck engaged to artificially inflate the vaccine's efficacy findings".

Another vaccine was exposed as flawed, in 2012, with a review of the Varicella (chickenpox) vaccination program in the U.S. This study concluded that the efficiency of Varicella had declined well below 80% by 2002 (journal Vaccine 12), if in fact it ever was as effective as the company claimed. Moreover, the Varicella vaccine has not proven to be cost-effective—as it increased the incidence of shingles—shifting medical costs from one ailment to another. It also failed to provide long-term protection from chicken pox, showing itself to be less effective than the natural immunity that existed in the general population, before the vaccine's introduction.

In 2012, British drug maker GlaxoSmithKline pled guilty to three counts of criminal misdemeanor relating to the prescription drugs Paxil, Wellbutrin, and Avandia, and agreed to pay $3 billion in fines. That payment was the largest fraud settlement in U.S. history, and the largest fine ever paid by a drug company.

A previous settlement (not quite that large) came from Pfizer, who paid $2.3 billion, in 2009, to settle similar fraud charges. Shortly thereafter, Abbott Laboratories paid $1.6 billion for wrongful marketing of the anti-seizure drug Depakote. (Abbott Labs had illegally promoted the drug to health care providers, for off-label use in seniors with dementia.)

Since 1997, 16 major drugs have been pulled from the North American market for injuring, or killing, patients. On top of that, every year, more than 15,000 people die in North America from over-the-counter drugs, like aspirin, Ibuprofen, and Tylenol.

According to a recent compilation of the top settlements by the drug industry, drug makers, over the past decade, have agreed to pay more than $11 billion in fines for illegal marketing. (www.fiercepharma.com)

The problem here is fines simply do not work; they have just become an additional price of doing business. By the time the fine is paid, immense profits have been made—well over and above the cost of any fines. Were the fines to include all profits made from the offending drugs, these companies might take the issue more seriously. Clearly, unnecessary loss of human life is not enough of a motivator for them to clean up their act.

STAY AWAY FROM DOCTORS

Not long ago, the most statistically dangerous thing you could do was get into a car, since the leading cause of death (until you reached the age when heart attack was a concern) was traffic accidents. Now the most dangerous thing you can do is to put yourself into the hands of the medical profession. Going to a doctor, clinic, hospital, or pharmacy, can literally endanger your life.

Let's look at a few more of the facts (within the U.S. medical system) discovered in that original Death by Medicine report.

- Adverse reactions to prescribed drugs = 2.2 million per year.

- Unnecessary antibiotics prescriptions (for viral infections) = 20 million per year.

- Unnecessary medical and surgical procedures = 7.5 million per year.

- Unnecessary hospitalization = 8.9 million per year.

These errors may not have killed anyone, but certainly did not help to prolong their lives—and most likely contributed to a worsening of long-term health, possibly hastening early death.

If only doctors had followed their ethical instincts, instead of selling out to the pharmaceutical industry, and violating their own Hippocratic Oath. ("I will prescribe regimens for the good of my patients according to my ability and my judgment and never do harm to anyone.") What a different world we would be living in now. Instead, we have a situation where those mandated to heal and protect us turn out to be the most dangerous threat to our wellbeing.

If you are reading this, I am probably preaching to the converted. You already know there is value to preventative medicine, in the form of dietary control, and nutritional supplements. And, you understand the necessity of taking responsibility for your own health, and the self-education that it requires.

This is all the more important now, as it gets more and more difficult to find a family doctor, here in Canada. Often, we end up seeing a stranger, at a walk-in clinic, who has no idea of our history. The doctor takes a quick stab at diagnosis, and sends us on our way with an antibiotic, or some other hastily prescribed drug. As we have just seen, the last thing we need are more casually prescribed medications.

PART ONE

ESSENTIAL SUPPLEMENTS

CHAPTER ONE

HOW THREE NUTRIENTS CAN HELP HEAL MOST AILMENTS

When not writing, or working on research and development, for NutriStart Vitamin Company, I work as a nutritional consultant in a vitamin store, which I have done (at one place or another) for over 30 years now. Over time, as my knowledge, and feedback from customers accumulated, I developed a unifying theory of illness. It presents not as a fully original theory (as the "leaky-gut" aspect of it is now well known), however, what is not well known is my approach. I have come to believe that a widespread deficiency in three key nutrients has caused an underlying problem (which is the link to many different illnesses), leaky gut being only one component of this problem.

WHAT CAUSES LEAKY GUT?

"Leaky gut" is just what it sounds like: a porous intestinal tract, no longer fully intact. Leaky gut is caused by a number of modern problems, the main one being candida yeast overgrowth.

Candida problems are most commonly caused by frequent antibiotic use, excessive sugars in the diet for long periods, mercury toxicity (usually from vaccines or dental fillings), and from birth control pills (via excessively high estrogen levels).

Another major cause of leaky gut is the consumption genetically modified canola oil, corn, and/or soybeans; the pesticide used on these crops (glyphosate, or "Roundup") is particularly damaging to the lining of the gut.

These crops were genetically modified to be resistant to glyphosate. Therefore, they can now take up, and retain, more of that pesticide—amounts that previously would have killed the plants. For the consumer, this means ingesting more of that pesticide than would have been possible before the genetic modification of these plants.

Ironically, many of those with celiac disease, and gluten-sensitivity, are consuming high amounts of corn and soy products (since they are gluten-free). If these products are made with genetically modified plants, then those food choices are actually contributing to worsening the underlying cause of the condition: damaged intestinal tract, and villi.

WHY IS LEAKY GUT SO DANGEROUS?

Since a leaky gut allows invasive compounds, and toxins to enter the bloodstream, this ailment is implicated in a wide range of health problems. Normally, these detrimental compounds would be neutralized by the liver, or excreted through normal channels of evacuation (feces, sweat, and urine). These compounds can be allergens, chemical toxins, or just large protein particles—all of which wreak havoc in the body by triggering allergic responses, inflammation, and even autoimmune conditions.

It is important to note here that inflammation, alone, is an underlying cause of many modern ailments—including heart disease, cancer, arthritis, and diabetes. Neurological problems, ranging from autism and anxiety, to depression and schizophrenia, have all been linked to protein particles—mostly from gluten and casein—entering the bloodstream, and making their way to the brain.

STANDARD APPROACH TO HEALING LEAKY GUT

Conventionally, natural health practitioners work to heal a leaky gut by restricting the diet—eliminating foods that trigger a negative response, as well as those foods that feed candida. Such offensive foods typically include wheat and/or grains containing gluten, cow's milk products (especially casein), and sugars (including tropical fruits, and all fruit juices).

The patient is also commonly advised to consume nutrients and supplements that help to heal gut lining. These include L-glutamine, licorice extracts in lozenge form (or DGL licorice, for those with high blood pressure), and N-acetyl-glucosamine. Other supplements often recommended include aloe vera juice (to reduce inflammation in the gut), and the herbs marshmallow and slippery elm—which soothe the irritated digestive tract, calming and coating it, allowing healing to occur.

The patient is usually also put on supplements designed to kill off candida overgrowth (to prevent further damage occurring), and given probiotics to counteract some of the damage caused by candida (and any antibiotics use).

BLOOD TYPE DIET

The above recommendations are all valid, however, in the case of autoimmune conditions, I believe it is also important that the patient follow the Blood Type Diet. ("Eat Right 4 Your Type", by Dr. Peter D'Adamo; www.dadamo.com) Essentially, the blood type diet defines your genetic heritage, and outlines which foods you are not genetically adapted to eating.

In the case of autoimmune conditions, particular protein particles called "lectins" enter the bloodstream, and cause an antibody response—often interpreted by the medical profession as an autoimmune condition.

I also recommend that anyone with a pre-diabetic, or inflammatory condition, follow the blood type diet closely—at least until health improvements occur. The blood type diet is of benefit here because certain foods contain lectins that cause an insulin spike and/or inflammation (in specific blood types). However, once the gut lining has thickened, the lectins are much less likely to enter the bloodstream, and one can broaden their diet again.

WHAT IS LEAKY GUT REALLY ABOUT?

Often overlooked by the conventional approach are underlying nutritional deficiencies that led to leaky gut in the first place. Also seldom considered (and the essence of my thesis), is that leaky gut is only one symptom of a general erosion of mucous membranes throughout the body.

Consider this: we are essentially a worm/tube with appendages. When the lining of the tube that separates us from the outside world is eroded, the outside world then has direct access to our bloodstream. Harmful substances enter blood through weak spots in our mucosal lining—whereas, when healthy, our mucosal lining filters out what is detrimental, and selectively allows in what is useful.

I believe this issue is the root cause of a wide range of ailments, and thus I have a protocol I administer to anyone with any condition relating to tubal erosion.

I have received amazing, positive feedback from those who follow this regimen, as they often reverse long-standing symptoms that no medical professional could help with.

MUCOUS MEMBRANE EROSION

So, for example, when sinuses lose their lining, they cannot filter out dander, dust, pollen, etc., and one is prone to allergies. Other symptoms can include post-nasal drip, nasal dryness, and eventually, sinus infections.

When the respiratory system loses its lining, we can be subject to bronchitis, lung infections, asthma, emphysema, and even throat problems that seem unexplainable.

When the stomach loses its lining ulcers can develop, and when the intestinal tract loses its lining the result is leaky gut—and all the aforementioned problems associated with that—as well as celiac disease, and food allergies.

When the genitourinary tract loses its lining, one is likely to have recurring bladder infections, kidney problems, interstitial cystitis, or vaginal dryness. The lining of the prostate thins and it becomes prone to infection, while thinning of the uterus can lead to endometriosis.

As well, part of the mucosal lining in many cases (sinuses, lungs, and intestinal tract) includes the fine "hairs" (villi, cilia) that keep those systems trapping, and expelling, foreign particles—again keeping them out of the bloodstream.

The loss of those fine hairs in the intestinal tract (villi) is the main cause of celiac disease, and a loss of those hairs in the lungs (cilia) leads to lung problems. However, when the cilia are healthy, the lungs are able to expel dust particles (and carbon particles from smog and smoke), as well as mucus (which also carries out toxins and waste), thus protecting the lungs from disease.

THREE CRITICAL NUTRIENTS

Now on to the big three nutritional deficiencies, which has led to this widespread erosion of mucosal lining: vitamins A, D, and iodine. All three of these nutrients are required by the body to build, maintain, and heal the mucous membranes. And, while a deficiency in any one is bad enough, a chronic deficiency in all three compounds the problem.

Each of these nutrients is necessary for a wide range of critical functions, over and above serving the mucous membranes. Thus, they all deserve to be used therapeutically by everyone, regardless of the current status of their mucosal lining.

VITAMIN A

Those who have read the first volume of Health Secrets, and/or who have read my early blogs, are already familiar with my unpopular stance in favor of vitamin A (though I am not alone in this belief). While it is generally believed by conventional medicine (and even by many naturopaths) that vitamin A can be dangerous and should be taken only in small amounts, this is blatantly false, and there is much evidence to prove it. This evidence is detailed in Volume One, and in my blogs on the subject (www.nutristart.com).

We are commonly deficient in vitamin A simply because we do not eat liver any more: the only appreciable source of vitamin A in the diet. Traditionally, humans ate organ meat frequently, unlike today when we mainly eat muscle meat—which is less nutritious, and harder to digest, than organs. A serving of cow liver (which my family ate at least once a week when I was growing up) contains about 40,000 IU of vitamin A. Many cultures still eat liver from a variety of sources (including chicken, goose, and lamb), but this now rare among North Americans.

Have a look at your multi-vitamin and see how much vitamin A it contains. Usually they contain no vitamin A, or at best, only a small amount (around 2,500 IU). However, most multi-vitamins do contain beta-carotene, to fulfill their vitamin A requirement. Unfortunately, most of them use synthetic beta-carotene, which is worthless as a supplement. Natural beta-carotene (whether from food or as a supplement) will convert into vitamin A, but you need to be in ideal health, and obtain a large amount of it, in order to produce sufficient vitamin A—especially if you are deficient.

Vitamin A deficiency is widespread in the developing world, and linked to night blindness, severe diarrhea, and lack of resistance to infection. I am convinced this deficiency is far more extensive in the Western world than we are led to believe, and one sign of this is the prevalence of sunglasses (more on this to follow).

VITAMIN D

Carcinomas represent 85% of all cancers, and they begin in the epithelial tissue—the tissue which lays on top of mucous membranes. Epithelial tissue lines the cavities, and surfaces of structures, throughout the entire body.

When scientific literature on vitamin D suggests that sufficient amounts may help prevent these types of cancers from occurring (as vitamin D helps regenerate epithelial tissue, and mucous membranes), it becomes obvious that maintaining a healthy mucosal structure is critical for one's well-being.

A study conducted by Creighton University School of Medicine (done between 2000 and 2005), showed a reduction in cancer risk of over 60%, from taking only 1,100 IU of vitamin D daily. (Reported in the June 8 online edition of the American Journal of Clinical Nutrition.)

Most people are massively deficient in vitamin D as a result of being told for decades that we only need 400 IU daily. In fact, if one is deficient in vitamin D, their body will make up to 10,000 IU in just half an hour of proper sunbathing. However, proper sunbathing is a little more complex than many assume.

In the temperate zones, only 4 months of the year provide enough sunshine to produce vitamin D. Even then, in order to produce vitamin D, one must have at least 50% body exposure, and must not shower or bath during the day. Washing (with soap and hot water) removes sebum (our natural body oil) from the skin, and sebum is required for the sun to produce our vitamin D. These days, nearly 80% of the population of India is deficient in vitamin D, so even living in a sunny climate is no indication you will produce sufficient D.

The links between vitamin D deficiency and health issues are practically countless, and include asthma, autism, diabetes, multiple sclerosis, and schizophrenia, to name a few. Therefore, vitamin D is perhaps the single most important nutrient one should take for optimal health—aside from its role in supporting mucous membranes.

IODINE

The third critical nutrient, absent from the modern diet, is iodine. (I will be brief here, since iodine has its own chapter.) This deficiency exists because we generally do not eat seaweed—the only reliable source of iodine in the diet. Of course, we have iodized table salt, but this salt is fortified with potassium iodide (not true iodine), and thus works mostly on the thyroid gland.

Iodine deficiency is linked to cognitive impairment, fibrocystic breast disease, heart disease, obesity, psychiatric disorders, and various forms of cancer. However, iodine is included here for its role in healing, and maintaining, mucous membranes.

OTHER NUTRIENTS FOR MUCOUS MEMBRANES

So, these are the big three, commonly deficient, critically required nutrients: vitamin A, vitamin D and iodine. And most ailments stem from long term (even generational) deficiencies of these three nutrients—not only because of their necessity for maintaining our mucous membranes, but also because of the wide range of bodily functions they are required for.

To a lesser degree, a fourth nutrient is also necessary for repairing mucous membranes (in some cases), and that is vitamin B-12. Vitamin B-12 deficiency is most commonly found among the elderly, strict vegetarians, those with blood type A or AB (middle aged, or older), and in those with severe intestinal disorders (IBS, celiac disease, Crohn's disease, or colitis).

Strict vegetarians, and vegans, enter into deficiency since true vitamin B12 is found only in animal foods. Blood types A and AB are (usually) genetically predisposed to low stomach acid, which also impedes B12 absorption. In cases of intestinal disorders, digestive malfunctions impede absorption of B-12 from the diet.

Chronic B-12 deficiency causes pernicious anemia, mood disorders, and neurological problems ranging from dementia to Parkinson's disease. In cases of B-12 deficiency, the supplement should be taken sublingually (under the tongue), or by injection, and preferably in the methylcobalamin form.

Other nutrients required for maintaining and repairing mucous membranes include, vitamin B2, zinc, and vitamin C. Vitamin C is required for collagen production—collagen being the "glue" that holds us together.

Most people I consult with (or those who read my blogs), are aware they need some basic nutritional support, outside of food. They are usually taking a multi-vitamin (which would include B2, and zinc), as well as extra vitamin C, so those bases are covered. What most people, even those with basic nutritional understanding, are not taking is the Big 3—and if they are, not in adequate amounts for our purposes.

THERAPEUTIC PROTOCOL

My protocol for healing mucosal membranes tends to the conservative side, and can take a few months to work fully. Doses of these nutrients can be higher, and perhaps results may occur faster, but this approach requires the guidance of a natural health professional. Nutrients may be much safer than drugs, but they are not without their own potential side effects (most often due to depleting other nutritional co-factors).

I always suggest my clients take the recommended supplement only five days a week—skipping two days. By taking a break two things are accomplished: the body is encouraged to use up any excess of a nutrient (especially in the case of non-water soluble nutrients, like minerals and fat-soluble vitamins), and we remind the body to store nutrients, since they will not be ingested consistently. Constantly taking a nutrient in high amounts, suggests to the body your environment is so rich in these nutrients it no longer needs to conserve them.

DOSING WITH VITAMIN A

Take 50,000 IU of vitamin A daily (with a meal containing fat) for 5 days, then 30,000 IU daily, until you do not squint on a sunny day. Squinting in the sunlight (outside of staring into the sun) is a feedback mechanism indicating vitamin A deficiency. Sensitivity to all bright lights indicates a more severe vitamin A deficiency (unless a medical condition is present). Other symptoms of vitamin A deficiency include dry eyes, and poor night vision.

After no longer squinting on sunny days, one can take 10,000 IU daily, five days a week (or 50,000 IU once a week). When sensitivity to light returns, I recommend going back to taking 3 or 4 pills (10,000 IU each) of vitamin A, until the problem recedes, and then roll back the dosage. I prefer naturally sourced vitamin A (from fish liver oil), however, synthetic vitamin A will also do the job (unlike synthetic beta-carotene), for those who are vegan.

DOSING WITH VITAMIN D

Take 10,000 IU of vitamin D, as drops (under the tongue), or soft gels (with a meal containing fat), for 5 days, then 5,000 IU daily, until the health issue alleviates. After that, take 3 to 5,000 IU daily. If you have been sunbathing properly, you can forgo ingesting vitamin D as a supplement for a few days thereafter. (For information on how to obtain a vitamin D test, and ideal blood levels of vitamin D, see my blogs, or e-book, on the subject, at www.nutristart.com.)

DOSING WITH IODINE

Japanese intake of iodine, from daily seaweed consumption, is between 1 to 3 mg daily, while here in the West, we are lucky to ingest 100 to 150 mcg daily.

For the purposes of rebuilding mucosal membrane, I recommend 3 mg of iodine, daily, either from nascent iodine, or from a mix of iodine and potassium iodide (such as Trophic Iodine, or Lugol's Solution). Iodine requires selenium as a co-factor, so, if you do not already take selenium (alone or in a multi-vitamin) it is a good idea to incorporate it into your nutritional regimen.

DOCTORS USED TO KNOW THIS

Recently, I was reading a booklet, written, in 1928, by pharmacists, for doctors who purchased their products. Here a pharmacist was enthusiastic about the new golden age of medicine soon to replace the ignorant superstitions of times previous. What I found fascinating was his enthusiasm for newly discovered vitamins, and how critical they were for growth, healing, and maintenance of good health.

Those nutrients that foretold a new golden age of healing were, interestingly enough, vitamins A and D, from cod liver oil, and iodine (as well as vitamins C, E, and the B vitamins). In fact, to quote from this booklet, "Dr. Douglas Harvey, at the Rowett Research Institute, Aberdeen, has reported that cod liver oil favorably influences the metabolism of iodine". This illustrates the medical profession at that time was aware of the synergistic interaction of these three nutrients. If doctors had only followed that course, there would be no need for books like this today.

The material covered in this chapter is not new information—it is just being rediscovered now. This is knowledge our ancestors had intuitively (i.e. eating organ meats; see www.westonaprice.org), before the advent of modern science, and the first rediscovery of it by the aforementioned medical professionals from 1928.

IODINE

The average person thinks little about iodine, assuming that it is required only for the thyroid gland, and is commonly available in our diet—or, at the very least, in our fortified table salt. But, iodine is far more deficient in the Western diet than is commonly believed, and proves to be one of the most important minerals required for good health.

Some iodine is found in seafood, but the highest amount is found in seaweeds, which are seldom eaten in the Western diet—thus the common deficiency. Most mammals require iodine for synthesizing thyroid hormones, and, to Western medicine, that is its only importance.

However, as we shall see, iodine performs many more functions than just supporting the thyroid gland, functions essential to good health. Even though the body of a healthy adult contains from 15 to 20 mg of iodine concentrated in thyroid tissue and hormones, the other 70% of the body's iodine is distributed in other tissues—including mammary glands, eyes, gastric mucosa, the cervix, and salivary glands.

IODINE AND THE THYROID

When one produces insufficient amounts of thyroid hormone, or when one is thyroid hormone-resistant, the result is "hypothyroidism" (underactive thyroid). When this occurs, normal metabolism cannot be maintained, and the ability to convert tyrosine (an amino acid) into the excitory neurotransmitters (dopamine, norepinephrine, and epinephrine), is impaired.

This can lead to a variety of symptoms, including cognitive dysfunction, extreme fatigue, goiter, mental slowing, depression, weight gain, and a slowing of the metabolic rate. One indication of a slowed metabolism, and one of the most common symptoms of hypothyroidism, is the sensation of feeling cold most of the time. This sensation occurs because the body cannot generate enough ATP (energy) molecules to keep the core temperature high enough to remain warm.

These days thyroid disease is extremely common, with anywhere from 10 to 40% of North Americans (depending on who you believe) having suboptimal thyroid function. People who are deficient in iodine, and also eat large amounts of foods containing goitrogens, can exacerbate symptoms of hypothyroidism.

Goitrogens are substances that interfere with the way the body uses iodine, and are found in certain plant foods, including soy, and cruciferous vegetables (cabbage, broccoli, cauliflower, Brussels sprouts, etc.). However, eating these foods cooked, rather than raw, will considerably reduce their role in inhibiting thyroid function. (For those consuming adequate amounts of iodine, eating foods containing goitrogens is of little concern.)

BENEFITS OF IODINE

Contrary to the myopic view of modern medicine, the benefits of iodine range far beyond simply supporting thyroid function. When the body has more iodine than the thyroid requires (that is, once the thyroid is saturated with it), iodine then begins to serve some other valuable functions. For example, iodine can remove toxic chemicals, including fluoride, bromide, lead, aluminum, and mercury, from our system. In fact, when initially increasing iodine intake, it is important to start slowly (and with gradual increases), or one can become ill from detoxifying too fast.

Iodine will also destroy cells contaminated with cancer and viruses, and can suppress an overactive immune system (in cases of autoimmune diseases). It strengthens the immune system, protects the stomach from abnormal bacteria growth, and can kill candida yeast overgrowth.

At the Center for Holistic Medicine, Doctors Abraham, Flechas, and Brownstein (iodine specialists) tested more than 4,000 patients. These people were taking iodine in daily doses ranging from 12.5 to 50 mg, and, in those with diabetes, up to 100 mg a day. These investigators found that "iodine does indeed reverse fibrocystic disease; their diabetic patients require less insulin; hypothyroid patients, less thyroid medication; symptoms of fibromyalgia resolve; and patients with migraine headaches stop having them". Clearly, iodine has many more functions than just supporting thyroid function.

BREAST HEALTH

Every cell, organ, and system in the human body needs iodine, but none more so than female breast tissue. Breast tissue has an even greater concentration of iodine than the thyroid. This leads some specialists to believe women with larger breasts may need more iodine than women with smaller breasts do. (And, women need more iodine than men.)

Research has proven iodine deficiency can lead to fibrocystic breast disease and/or ovarian cysts. Therefore, in the field of natural healing, iodine treatment is used to reduce uterine fibroids; indeed, one of the early conventional medical treatments for severe fibroids was to paint iodine on the abdomen, over the area where the fibroids were located.

In fact, all reproductive disorders can be caused (or worsened by) iodine deficiency. Iodine deficiency is also linked to a variety of cancers including breast, ovarian, prostate, stomach, testicular, thyroid, and uterine. (1)

On a personal note, a friend of mine had been plagued with painful lumps and cysts in her breasts for her entire adult life. After finding out about iodine and breast health, she started taking high doses of Lugol's Iodine Solution, working up to 60 mg of iodine/iodide daily. She fully cured this condition, and now faithfully takes iodine, though at a much lower dosage.

Iodine is also necessary for optimal functioning of a number of body systems, including gastric mucosa, salivary glands, oral mucosa, and arterial walls. Here I want to touch briefly on the importance of iodine for rebuilding, and maintaining, mucous membranes.

MUCOUS MEMBRANE

Even if it had no other benefits, the function of iodine in maintaining the integrity of mucous membranes would be reason enough to supplement with it. This function is one reason potassium iodide (synthetic iodine) used to be prescribed as an expectorant—although few doctors remember that now.

The necessity of iodine for maintaining mucous membranes was originally brought to my attention by two clients I consulted with. Both told me they avoided surgery for post-nasal drip, simply by adding a moderate amount (about 1 mg) of iodine to their nutritional regimen.

During my research, I discovered there was a time (before the advent of pharmaceutical drugs) when a medical professional baffled by an ailment simply gave the patient more iodine. In those times, hospitals also effectively cleaned with diluted iodine (something that could now help combat "superbugs"—antibiotic-resistant bacteria), and it was widely used for a multitude of purposes. I believe it is time for the medical profession to rediscover this inexpensive miracle worker.

IODINE DEFICIENCY

Over the last 30 to 40 years, the intake of iodine has dropped by over 50% in the U.S. (which can be extrapolated to Canada as well). During this same period, we have seen increases in the rates of diabetes, high blood pressure, obesity, breast and thyroid cancer, and thyroid disorders—all of which, some experts believe, are directly related to iodine deficiency. (2)

According to the World Health Organization (WHO), 72% of the world's population is iodine deficient, and, according to another source, 96% of the U.S. population is also deficient. (3)

In areas of the world where the diet lacks sufficient iodine (typically areas where no marine foods are consumed), iodine deficiency manifests primarily as hypothyroidism.

However, more than just a cause of thyroid malfunction, iodine deficiency is the leading cause of intellectual disability in the world—a result of infants, or small children, lacking this vital mineral. (Iodine deficiency, and hypothyroidism, in adults may cause temporary mental slowing, but not permanent intellectual disability.)

Iodine deficiency is widespread due to seaweed being the only reliable source of this mineral in the diet (with seafood coming in a distant second). It seems only people who live near the sea eat seaweed regularly, and in the West (even if we do live near the sea) seaweed is only consumed occasionally—usually at a Japanese restaurants.

The modern approach of adding iodine to table salt has (for the most part) eliminated the problem of slowed mental development in the Western nations, but severe iodine deficiency is still a serious health issue in the developing world. And, iodized table salt has by no means solved the whole problem of this deficiency, even in areas where it is regularly consumed.

IODIZED SALT

The problem with iodized table salt (which has fallen out of favor with health-minded people) is that it is fortified with potassium *iodide*, not true iodine. Potassium iodide, a synthetic form of iodine, primarily serves the thyroid gland, whereas the body has receptor sites for iodine everywhere. While potassium iodide supports thyroid function, and protects the thyroid against radiation, true iodine does that and so much more (as discussed above).

In North America, not long ago, our iodine intake was much higher, due to the commercial use of iodine as a dough conditioner. Back then, each slice of bread would offer almost the full RDI of iodine. However, in the early 1970s, commercial bakeries turned to using bromide instead of iodine, at which point that ready source of iodine was lost. Perhaps even more concerning, bromide competes with iodine in the body—effectively blocking iodine uptake (as does fluoride). Iodized table salt also contains high chloride levels, which can further inhibit iodine uptake.

There is another reason synthetic iodine is a poor substitute for the naturally occurring form—iodine found in food will contain its own co-factors for absorption (including copper, tin, zinc, manganese, magnesium, and selenium). All nutrients depend on other nutrients for assimilation so, for example, too much zinc will deplete copper, and vice versa.

Therefore, I recommend those who are taking iodine as an isolated supplement also take a trace mineral supplement, or eat seaweed, on a regular basis. This ensures they are acquiring the necessary co-factors required to properly assimilate iodine, and to prevent depletion of any co-factor nutrients that high iodine levels may draw upon.

The trace mineral supplement I suggest is Concentrace Mineral Drops. This liquid is solar-evaporated inland sea water, with the sodium removed, and it has a mineral profile similar to seaweed, and human blood.

The thyroid gland only requires about 70 mcg of iodine daily, in order to synthesize necessary amounts of thyroid hormones T4 and T3. However, the Recommended Daily Intake (RDI) of iodine is

150 mcg per day, which at least acknowledges that iodine has other functions to perform—over and above supporting the thyroid gland. Unfortunately, the RDI is not acknowledging the amount of iodine necessary to support these other functions.

IODINE MADNESS

For experimental purposes, I have ingested as much as 100 mg of iodine, building up the dose over a few weeks (having started at 6 mg). This clearly flies in the face of the RDI of 150 mcg (1000 mcg in one milligram). So, I took over 600 times the recommended amount, and while this may sound ludicrous, there is a certain amount of method to my madness.

My interest in iodine began with an article in the local paper about a doctor recommending unusually high amounts of iodine to his patients. This physician, Dr. David Derry, went on to self-publish a book called "Breast Cancer and Iodine" (Trafford Press, available on Amazon), based on the thesis that Japanese iodine intake is about twenty times more than in the West, and, as a result, their rates of breast cancer are far less. At this time, the belief was the Japanese daily intake of iodine was between 12 mg and 18 mg. (Their high iodine intake is due to the large amounts of seaweed they consume, on top of a diet high in seafoods.)

However, as I mentioned in Health Secrets: Volume One, we must stay on top of new information related to health issues, since, what appears to be valid one year is often revealed to be wrong, or incomplete, in following years. Some may feel this to be unscientific, but true science is a field of proposing theories, and following up in later years to see if they work, and hold true.

JAPANESE IODINE INTAKE

In my original blog on iodine, I stated that the Japanese acquire 12 to 18 mg of iodine a day, based on what Dr. Derry (as well as other alternative sources) maintained. At least I took that amount, and much more, for quite some time, to test the waters before I encouraged anyone to dive in. I experienced no obvious negative side effects from this experiment, and eventually I went back to taking a modicum of iodine (about 1-3 mg daily).

Nevertheless, the idea that daily Japanese iodine intake is 12–18 mg has now been called into question. Dr. Alan Gaby, MD, in an article published in Townsend Letter (Aug/Sept 2005), pointed out that the claim of such high iodine intake amongst the Japanese was based on a misinterpretation of a 1967 paper (J Clin Endocrinol Metab 1967;27:638-47), analyzing seaweed consumption in Japan.

The Japanese consume on average almost five grams of seaweed daily. However, when the researchers tried to determine the amount of iodine this provided, they made the mistake of basing their numbers on the dry weight of seaweed, not the cooked, wet, amount consumed. This led to the idea that the Japanese consumed huge amounts of iodine, when in fact a 2008 study showed average iodine intake to be around 1.2 mg per day—down from an average of 1.7 mg per day in 1986. (Thyroid 2008:18:667)

Another inquiry into Japanese iodine intake combined information from dietary records, food surveys, urine iodine analysis, and seaweed iodine content. This study estimated the Japanese iodine intake averaged from 1 to 3 mg per day. (4)

This line of inquiry is important to me because I believe daily optimal intake of any given nutrient should be within the range of normal human dietary patterns. While nutrients can be used therapeutically at high levels (almost like drugs), once the therapy is over, we need to know what is a reasonable amount to continue ingesting. So, in this case, I am happy to consume, and recommend, from 1 to 3 mg of iodine daily (5 days a week).

IODINE AND PREGNANCY

Of course, the Japanese consume seaweed generationally, which is to say, one's mother ate seaweed every day, and her mother did so as well. This means a healthy amount of iodine is passed on to the offspring, giving them a good storage level to begin life with.

It is acknowledged in the West that pregnant and nursing women require more iodine than normal. In the U.S., pregnant women are advised to consume 220 micrograms of iodine daily, and those who are breastfeeding require 290 mcg a day. Being well aware iodine is critical for the healthy development of a baby's brain and nervous system, medical authorities recommend these higher amounts for pregnant and nursing mothers.

In iodine-deficient areas of the world, studies have proven supplementation with iodine before or during early pregnancy will prevent cretinism, increase birth weight, reduce rates of infant mortality, and increase cognitive developmental scores in young children by 10–20%. (5)

A study published in The Lancet medical journal (2013), showed even mild iodine deficiency during pregnancy could be a factor in a child's mental development. The researchers studied 1,040 pregnant women (in England), and eight years later followed up by testing their children's IQ scores.

They discovered the women who were mildly to moderately deficient in iodine during pregnancy, were more likely to have children with lower IQ scores at age 8—particularly verbal and reading scores. (6) In fact, research has shown mothers with low levels of iodine are also more likely to have an autistic child. (7)

DR. DERRY

Back to Dr. David Derry, who triggered my interest in iodine therapy. Dr. Derry used a thyroid test on his patients, more subtle in nature than what is commonly used in the medical field. (I continually see people who feel they may have an under-active thyroid, but have tested, by conventional medical thyroid tests, at acceptable levels.)

Unfortunately, it appears the conventional thyroid test only reveals serious problems with thyroid health. Some alternative practitioners maintain that, by the time your thyroid malfunction registers on a modern thyroid test, you will have already lost almost 70% of your thyroid function—leading inevitably to a prescription for Synthroid. While this synthetic hormone may serve the function of keeping the thyroid working, it is no substitute for providing iodine, nor does it fulfill the many other functions that iodine serves in the body.

The test Dr. Derry recommended for detecting subtle thyroid malfunction involves placing a thermometer under your arm, first thing in the morning, and remaining quiet, and still, for about 15 minutes. After this length of time, you can take your reading: a temperature of 97.6 degrees Fahrenheit, or lower, consistently for 5 days, indicates an under-active thyroid.

LUGOL'S SOLUTION

Dr. Derry recommended his patients use a compound called Lugol's Solution, an inexpensive liquid iodine product, which provides 6 mg of iodine per drop (at a 5% solution). The most commonly available version of Lugol's Solution contains 5% iodine, and 10% potassium iodide.

Lugol's Solution, named after the French physician, J. Lugol, was first produced in 1829, and is a solution comprised of elemental iodine, and potassium iodide, in water.

It is available over the counter in Canada (usually through a Compounding Pharmacy), however in the U.S. (since 2007) the DEA has regulated Lugol's Solution—and all iodine solutions containing greater than 2.2% iodine—since it is used in the illegal production of methamphetamine. (Though, in the U.S., one may still buy small amounts of iodine solution—up to 1oz—without a prescription.)

Dr. Derry reported many satisfied patients—their energy level returned to normal, their weight balanced out, and a disappearance of breast problems (such as cysts, and fibrocystic breast disease) occurred. However, when he lost his license to be a general practitioner (though he was still allowed to practice as a surgeon), none of these patients were able to testify at his inquiry. This is all hearsay from my perspective (never having met the man), and to be fair, it was claimed by the medical association that there were a couple of adverse reactions to his iodine protocol, initiating the inquiry in the first place.

I am enough of a conspiracy theorist to believe an inexpensive solution to thyroid problems (such as iodine) is simply not the kind of business generator a prescription solution is—especially one that you need to take for the rest of your life (such as Synthroid). The attack on Dr. Derry occurred only after the article in the newspaper highlighted his unique, and inexpensive, approach to thyroid issues.

Anecdotal information on the use of Lugol's Solution indicates its multiple applications. Examples include treating simple food poisoning (6 drops in one cup of water), salmonella (6 drops in water, 4 times daily, for 3 days), and colds and flu (6 drops in water, 3 times over a 24 hr period). Diluted Lugol's can be sprayed onto infected tonsils (no dilution specifications, nor time frame was given), and, I have personally used a few drops of undiluted Lugol's Solution topically, to effectively treat abscesses, and dental infections.

IODINE SUPPLEMENTS

In multivitamins, iodine usually occurs in the form of synthetic potassium iodide, while most liquid iodine supplements are a mix of iodine, and potassium iodide. However, liquid iodine supplements usually contain a lower percentage of both forms of iodine than Lugol's Solution. For example, Lugol's Solution (5%) provides 6 mg of mixed iodine/iodide in one drop, whereas Trophic liquid iodine contains one tenth as much per drop. These weaker forms work well for most people, but some who are in poor health achieve better results with the form of iodine known as "nascent" iodine.

Nascent iodine is a pure iodine (no iodide) in its atomic form, and is unlike other iodine products, which have a more complex molecular structure. This makes it the most assimilable form of iodine, especially valuable for those with difficulty absorbing nutrients.

Nascent iodine is recognized by the body as the same form of iodine that is received by the thyroid. It is absorbed effortlessly, and is taken up by all the cells, not just the thyroid. And, whereas prescription medications, containing thyroid hormones, take over the thyroid's job, nascent iodine nutritionally rebuilds the thyroid so it can function on its own.

Unlike most natural iodine supplements, nascent iodine is derived from inland minerals, rather than from seaweed. Therefore, it contains no naturally occurring bromide, which some people are allergic to.

When taking iodine in liquid form, do not put it into a beverage high in vitamin C (such as orange juice), since vitamin C will chemically transform iodine into iodide, reducing its benefits.

It should be mentioned that, according to one iodine "expert", nascent iodine "will not saturate body tissues and has not been proven to detox halides (bromide, fluoride, chloride), and mercury, as other forms have" ("The Guide to Supplementing with Iodine" by Stephanie Burst N.D.).

Most of the anecdotal feedback on detoxifying with iodine is based on using Lugol's Solution. Since we have no clear scientific evidence concerning the detoxification aspects of iodine/iodide, I would suggest using Lugol's Solution, if one is attempting to detoxify heavy metals and/or bromides.

For those who do not want to take their iodine in liquid form, there is a tablet called Iodoral, which is equal to two drops of Lugol's Solution (12 mg).

FIBROMYALGIA

Dr. John Lowe is a specialist with extensive experience in treating patients with both thyroid disease and fibromyalgia. He is the

Director of Research for the Fibromyalgia Research Foundation, and the author of The Metabolic Treatment of Fibromyalgia.

Fibromyalgia is a condition with symptoms of severe musculoskeletal pain, and heavy fatigue. Dr. Lowe believes thyroid dysfunction is a factor in fibromyalgia, and the conventional medical thyroid test is useless for making either diagnosis.

Thus, one can have a thyroid test appear normal to a doctor, and still have a deficiency of thyroid hormone. Some people are resistant to thyroid hormone, in much the same manner that a diabetic can be insulin resistant. Thyroid hormone resistance means that a patient needs higher than "normal" amounts of thyroid hormone, in order to maintain proper metabolism and good health.

This is confirmed somewhat by the fact many thyroid patients who have "normal" Thyroid-Stimulating Hormone (TSH) levels, while taking thyroid hormone replacement, find that over time, they begin to develop joint and muscle pains, and arthritis-like symptoms—symptoms much akin to those of fibromyalgia.

Dr. Lowe recommends treating fibromyalgia with thyroid hormone until symptoms improve, and he has reported a high rate of success among his patients that follow this protocol. Dr. Lowe typically starts hypothyroid patients with a natural desiccated thyroid product; this natural form of thyroid hormones has proven to be more effective than using synthetic thyroid hormones.

Here is a list of the symptoms of hypothyroidism and thyroid hormone resistance, which are also symptoms of fibromyalgia: anxiety, bowel disturbances, chronic fatigue, cold intolerance, depression, dry skin, hair and mucous membranes, headaches, numbness and tingling, poor memory and concentration, sleep disturbance, stiffness, and widespread pain and tenderness. Clearly enough crossover symptoms to support the thesis of Dr. Lowe.

FOOD SOURCES OF IODINE
Seaweed (including dulse, kelp, nori, kombu, and wakame) is

simply the best food source of iodine, but it is highly variable in its content. The iodine content of seaweed can vary from 16 mcg to almost 3,000 mcg per gram, depending on the variety, and the time and location of harvest.

Kelp is the richest food source of iodine with 1 tablespoon of powder providing about 2000 mcg (2 mg) of iodine. Other seaweeds are much lower in iodine: 1 tablespoon of arame contains about 730 mcg of iodine, 1 tablespoon of hiziki contains about 780 mcg of iodine, and 1 tablespoon of wakame contains about 80 mcg of iodine.

You should be aware that, if the water the seaweed grows in is contaminated (e.g. heavy metals, radiation), the seaweed will be contaminated as well. Currently, there is concern that the radioactive water issuing from the collapsed Fukushima nuclear plant will contaminate seaweed (as well as fish). Since the Atlantic contains far less radiation than the Pacific Ocean, I almost exclusively use Atlantic dulse. (One gram of dulse provides about 150 to 300 mcg of iodine.)

In his book, Spiritual Nutrition, Dr. Gabriel Cousens concludes that, even though dulse has a lower iodine content than kelp, it may prove the better choice for supplying iodine. He holds this belief because dulse contains more manganese than kelp, and manganese is an important nutrient for the absorption and function of iodine in the body. (Dulse is also high in the trace mineral lithium, which is important for a healthy mood and mental state.)

Other sources of iodine:

- Seafood: 3oz of baked cod provides about 99 mcg; 100 grams of lobster provides about 100 mcg of iodine.

- Dairy products (partly due to the use of iodine feed supplements, and iodine-based sanitizing agents used in the dairy industry): 1 cup plain, low-fat yogurt provides about 75 mcg.

- Eggs: 1 large egg provides about 12 mcg.

- Cranberries: 4 oz provides about 400 mcg of iodine.

- Strawberries: 1 cup provides about 13 mcg of iodine.

- Navy beans: ½ cup provides about 32 mcg of iodine.

- Potatoes with skins: 1 medium baked potato provides about 60 mcg of iodine.

- Human breast milk (if the mother is not deficient), and infant formulas.

Iodine is found in other fruits, grains, and vegetables as well, though the amount (as with those options listed above) varies, depending on the iodine content of the soil, fertilizer use, and irrigation practices. Obviously, when these fruits and vegetables are organically grown they will contain more iodine than commercially grown products, and, the iodine content of meat and dairy products will likewise be affected by the iodine contained in foods the animals consume.

According to Canadian Dieticians, 1 teaspoon of iodized table salt contains 380 mcg of iodine (as iodide). However, the majority of salt intake in North America is obtained from processed foods, and commercial food manufacturers use non-iodized salt in their products (including things like canned soup).

If you are trying to avoid conventional table salt, but are worried about not consuming adequate iodine, Himalayan salt offers an alternative. Half a gram of Himalayan salt provides about 250 mcg of iodine. The other advantage of Himalayan salt over conventional table salt is it contains all the minerals found in seawater (much akin to the ratio of minerals found in human blood).

As well, Himalayan salt contains only 35% sodium (unlike refined table salt, which contains 98% sodium) with the balance being magnesium, potassium, and all the other trace minerals. Celtic sea salt (or any other unrefined sea salt) will also provide a similar amount of iodine as Himalayan salt (and the same percentage of sodium), along with the other minerals.

IODINE TOXICITY

When using iodine supplements at high doses (over 5 mg daily) for a long period of time, watch for possible symptoms of over-active thyroid. Such symptoms include anxiety, insomnia, diarrhea, high pulse rate, high blood pressure, rapid weight loss, sensitive or bulging eyes, and vision disturbances.

Some people are more sensitive to iodine than others, and thus are more likely to have side effects, even at low dose. Also, some people with autoimmune thyroid disease may experience adverse effects with iodine amounts normally considered safe for the general population.

At the Center for Holistic Medicine (which specializes in iodine therapy), the most common adverse effect they report is a metallic taste in the mouth, and/or acne. Acne (in this case), they believe, is actually due to a detoxification reaction.

Anecdotal information suggests one way to tell if we are taking too much iodine is an increase in nasal moisture (i.e., constantly "running" nose). If this symptom occurs, cease taking iodine until your nasal moisture levels return to normal.

Medical literature indicates that iodine toxicity occurs most often from topical application, usually in a hospital setting. When used internally, the dangerous aspects of iodine are modified in the stomach, making it very difficult to overdose on orally ingested iodine.

Acute iodine toxicity occurs somewhere around 2 grams, per day (ISMP Canada Safety Bulletin. 2011; 11(7):1-3). In fact, there is one incident in the medical casebooks where a fellow mistook his aunt's liquid iodine preparation in the fridge (which she used for her rheumatism) for iced tea. He ingested 15,000 mg (15 g) of iodine over a short period, and while he had symptomatic swelling of the face, neck and mouth, as well as transient cardiac arrhythmias, he recovered uneventfully with no residual problems.

In a study of 1,365 women who were treated with moderately high doses of iodine, for fibrocystic breast disease, 11% showed side effects that included acne, agitation, nausea, diarrhea, thinning hair, skin rash, and headaches. These women received between 3 and 6 mg of iodine per day. (8)

I will mention again that iodine requires certain co-factors. Often in these studies, researchers use isolated iodine without the other necessary nutrients required for proper assimilation—and still, side effects are uncommon. And, really, 11% adverse reaction is not that high, compared with many pharmaceutical drugs.

Here is the conclusion of Dr. Gaby (author of revised Japanese iodine intake article): 3 to 6 mg of iodine is a therapeutic dose (which may be useful for treating fibrocystic breast disease), and higher doses may be advised for short periods, for the purposes of destroying intestinal pathogens.

THOSE WITH THYROID PROBLEMS

Mary Shomon, one of the leading educators in the U.S. on thyroid health (www.thyroid-info.com), warns those with thyroid diseases not to load up on iodine, or iodine-rich seaweeds. In someone without iodine deficiency, excessive iodine supplementation can actually worsen a pre-existing thyroid condition or trigger further thyroid dysfunction. She believes, for those with serious thyroid malfunction, the trick is to consume just the right amount of iodine—not too much, nor too little.

In such cases, it is ideal to take an iodine test—the type that measures the amount of iodine excreted in urine. The "urine iodine challenge test", available through an open-minded doctor, or naturopath, requires you to collect your urine for 24 hours, and then send the sample off to a lab. There they calculate your iodine level, based on the amount of iodine spilling into your urine. This test is the most accurate way to assess your iodine status.

While hypothyroidism is very common in the West (due in part to inefficient thyroid testing), actually treating it with iodine seems only to work if the individual is deficient. Otherwise, supplementing with iodine may worsen symptoms. For example, one Japanese study looked at the frequency of iodine-induced hypothyroidism. In this study, 33 people with hypothyroidism—25 women, 8 men, from 21 to 77 years old—stopped taking any iodine-containing drugs or foods (especially seaweed products), for up to 2 months. More than half the people in this study recovered from primary hypothyroidism after restricting iodine intake.

However, some specialists (www.iodineonmymind.com) believe it was the consumption of high amounts of iodine found in seaweed, causing the problem—not iodine per se. They believe this problem occurs because seaweed is high in bromide. There is 1400 times more bromide in seawater than iodine, and bromide is a goitrogen (a substance that suppresses the function of the thyroid).

One naturopath (Alan Christianson, ND) has found patients taking very high levels of iodine tend to manifest symptoms including multinodular goiter, Graves' disease, and Hashimoto's thyroiditis. In one of these cases, the patient was taking 50 mg of iodine daily (which even I think is excessive). High levels of iodine should only be taken for a short time-period, and then rolled back to a maintenance level.

This naturopath also noted, some patients on high-dose iodine had no adverse symptoms, and some patients not taking iodine still develop thyroid disease. However, he maintains, "the data that high-dose iodine can help fibrocystic breast disease is clear".

As I have mentioned before (and as is the belief in the field of "orthomolecular nutrition"), isolated nutrients can be used like drugs, at high doses for short periods, to a great positive effect. However, it is illogical to think that high doses are going to be valuable over the long run. (Although Dr. Abram Hoffer was still taking 3 to 4 grams of niacin daily at the time of his death—near the age of 90—so even this theory has its exceptions).

The iodine information becomes more clouded by statistics indicating Japanese in coastal areas, who consume high levels of iodine (via seaweed), have higher rates of thyroid disease than North Americans. Yet, Japanese populations who have low iodine intakes (from 100–200 mcg daily), have higher rates of thyroid problems too. Again, this may be due to the high bromide levels found in seaweed.

Information from WHO (based on tracking iodine-fortified salt levels around the world), seems to indicate that consuming higher than 600 mcg for long periods is linked to higher rates of both hypothyroidism, and hyperthyroidism (over-active thyroid). Of course, since synthetic potassium iodide is used to fortify table salt (not a natural source of iodine, and lacking co-factors), the results may be suspect.

HOW MUCH IODINE TO TAKE

Are there any easy answers? Not really. It appears both insufficient, and excessive, amounts of iodine can be problematic. Dr. Christianson believes a safe daily intake is 150 mcg, and occasionally 1,000 mcg (1 mg) is tolerable. I, among others, believe that short-term, high levels of iodine (for specific therapeutic purposes), can be of value. However, therapeutic doses should be taken for only a brief period—ideally with the guidance of a health professional.

I believe we can safely ingest amounts of iodine in the range of what the Japanese diet contains (1 to 3 mg daily)—if we consume it as a food (i.e. seaweed, if one is not allergic to bromide). If, however, we choose to get this amount of iodine in supplement form, then we should also ensure we consume adequate amounts of the cofactors iodine requires. As always, I recommend skipping supplementation a couple of days every week, to provide the body a chance to use up any excess iodine.

Considering the recent Fukushima disaster, we should also be aware of the very real potential for other nuclear power plant meltdowns. Thus, we will want to keep our iodine levels relatively high, in case of such a tragedy occurring in our vicinity. Iodine-131 is a component of nuclear fallout, and is particularly dangerous, owing to the tendency of the thyroid gland to concentrate any form of iodine.

Radioactive iodine is stored in the thyroid for periods longer than this isotope's half-life of eight days. For this reason, if people are about to be exposed to significant amounts of radioactive iodine, they are instructed to take high amounts of potassium iodide. This will block the thyroid from up-taking radioactive iodine—however, even better, is to have the thyroid already pre-saturated with healthful iodine.

DRUG INTERACTIONS

Iodine supplements have the potential to interact with several types of medications, so those taking such medications should discuss their iodine intake with a healthcare professional.

Anti-thyroid medications, such as methimazole (Tapazole), are used to treat hyperthyroidism. Taking high doses of iodine with anti-thyroid medications can have an additive effect, and could cause hypothyroidism.

Angiotensin-converting enzyme (ACE) inhibitors, such as benazepril (Lotensin), and lisinopril (Prinivil and Zestril), are used to treat high blood pressure. Taking potassium iodide with ACE inhibitors can increase the risk of hyperkalemia (elevated blood levels of potassium).

Potassium-sparing diuretics, such as spironolactone (Aldactone) and amiloride (Midamor), when combined with potassium iodide, can also increase the risk of hyperkalemia.

The thyroid gland needs iodine to synthesize hormones T4 and T3, but when Synthroid is used, we are ingesting an end-product hormone, and bypassing the natural process in the body. Long-term use of thyroid hormone medications is associated with depletion of thyroid and tissue iodine levels, as well as increased rates of cancer. Therefore, anyone taking thyroid medications should talk to a pharmacist about the safe amount of iodine to take along with their medication.

A WORD ABOUT SELENIUM

As mentioned above, there are a few co-factors that iodine requires for proper absorption and assimilation. These include copper, tin, zinc, manganese, magnesium, and selenium. Of these, selenium is the most important. Selenium (along with iodine) is critically important for T4 to T3 conversion in the liver, and it is important to supplement with it for any kind of thyroid problem. High levels of iodine, in the absence of selenium, can damage the thyroid gland (often felt as a sore throat).

Selenium plays a critical role in the production of glutathione, the body's most powerful antioxidant. Glutathione is necessary, in this case, because during the production of thyroid hormones, hydrogen peroxide is also produced. This internally generated hydrogen peroxide is a form of free radical, and is neutralized by glutathione. In turn, an excess of selenium increases the body's need for iodine, and deficiency will occur when the diet is high in selenium, and low in iodine.

Usually it is desirable to acquire between 100 and 200 mcg of selenium daily—an amount found in many multivitamin products.

When using high amounts of iodine (milligrams), it is also beneficial to supplement with vitamin C (at least 500mg three times daily, but not at the same time as the iodine consumption), magnesium (600mg daily in divided doses), and a B-complex. These ancillary nutrients work to both help the body absorb iodine, and to aid in removing toxins motivated out of the cells by the high iodine intake.

TOPICAL IODINE

Externally, iodine is commonly used as an antiseptic, for disinfecting drinking water, and is used medically to prevent surgical wound infections. (Topically, tincture of iodine kills 90% of bacteria in 90 seconds.)

Knowing these benefits, I tried topical iodine to treat a skin condition I once had (roseacea). I mixed 9 drops of Lugol's Solution, into two of ounces of aloe vera juice, and sprayed it onto my face morning and night, effectively curing my roseacea (after a few months). I have also used Lugol's Solution topically to disinfect and treat abscesses (on the gums), boils, cysts, and fungal infections.

Ever since the discovery of iodine by Bernard Courtois (in 1811), iodine has widely been used topically, for the prevention and treatment of all manner of skin infections and wounds. Iodine is recognized as an effective broad-spectrum bactericide—also effective against yeasts, molds, fungi, viruses, and protozoans.

The problem with topical use of iodine tincture is it stains the skin, and can irritate damaged tissue. As well, it will enter the bloodstream, raising unpredictable levels of iodine in the body.

In 1955, a new liquid form of iodine (Providone) was invented. This new form demonstrated powerful antibacterial activity, but proved to be less potentially toxic than conventional tincture of iodine, was non-irritating, and did not stain.

Providone also has a longer lasting antiseptic effect than conventional tincture of iodine, due to its slow absorption through skin. Even more impressive is that bacteria do not develop a resistance to Providone—although this would also hold true for all forms of topical iodine.

Providone is produced in different forms (spray, ointment, etc.), ranging from 7 to 12% iodine content. It is commonly used in hospitals as a topical antiseptic, to treat and prevent infection found in abrasions, blisters, burns, cuts, ulcers, and wounds. Providone is also used as a surgical scrub, for pre-operative and post-operative skin cleansing, and in gynecology for vaginitis associated with candidal, trichomonal, or mixed infections.

For our purposes, there are now commercially available diluted forms of Providone (containing 10% Providone) that are available without a prescription. These include Equate, Wokadine, or Betadine—the latter being the most commonly available version.

Anecdotal information on the use of Betadine topically (www. earthclinic.com) suggests a variety of uses, aside from the obvious disinfecting properties listed above. Some people have used Betadine to treat bald spots on the scalp, believing that such spots are are a result of fungus, which iodine kills. Others use it to harden fingernails by dipping them in Betadine iodine once a day for one week, then once a week for 3 to 4 weeks. Another reported use is the removal of moles and skin tags, by rubbing Betadine on them daily, for about a week.

Iodine is often used in third world countries as a field treatment for contaminated water. And, Betadine can also be used for water purification in emergencies (although this technique has not been approved by the EPA). By adding 8 drops of Betadine to a liter of water, it is believed most pathogens will be killed within 10 minutes (though it may not be effective against cryptosporidia).

BROMIDES

At this point, I am going to cover the subject of bromides, which, while it may be better suited to the chapter on Xenoestrogens, is here because of its special relationship to iodine.

Synthetic bromide is prevalent in our environment, and can wreak havoc on the thyroid. Moreover, this chemical (like many others covered in the Xenoestrogens chapter) is an endocrine disruptor, meaning it negatively affects our hormones, reproductive functions, and fetal and childhood development.

Bromide is a derivative of bromine (an element in the periodic table) which, when it is reacted with a metal, forms a "bromide". Bromide can occur naturally, most often in seawater, seafood, and seaweed, and the body can tolerate this form, in small amounts.

A bromate is another bromine-based chemical, sometimes found as a contaminant in water, and is considered a carcinogen. When fresh water contains high amounts of bromide (either naturally occurring, or from groundwater contamination), and when that water

K.W. PETERS

is treated with ozone (as with many bottled waters), the ozone can react with bromide ions in the water to produce bromate.

Other bromated forms of bromine are sodium bromate, used mostly in dyes (for fabric and hair), and potassium bromate, used mostly as a dough conditioner for baked goods. For our purposes, all forms of bromine, including bromate and bromide, as well as a few other chemical variations (mentioned further on) are toxic, and to be avoided as much as possible.

Bromide is known as a halogen (a group in the periodic table, which includes chlorine, fluorine, and iodine), and easily slips into the same receptors in the body that iodine normally occupies. Primarily it will occupy the iodine receptors in the thyroid, inhibiting hormone production, and causing hypothyroidism. As well, if we are exposed to, or ingest, large amounts of bromide (and/or chlorine and fluoride), other areas of the body requiring iodine, will also fail to retain the iodine we consume (since those receptors will already be occupied).

In the 19th and early 20th century, potassium bromide was used as a medication—given it had sedative properties. As late as 1975, Bromo-Seltzer (used to treat stomach upset, headaches, and hangovers) contained bromide. However, around that time, the FDA required most medications remove bromide—being aware by then it had toxic properties. Although, apparently not toxic enough for the FDA to entirely outlaw bromides.

AVOIDING BROMIDES

■ Methyl bromide is a broad-spectrum pesticide used in the control of pest insects, nematodes, weeds, pathogens, and rodents. It is also used as a fungicide to treat soil, and for structural fumigation. Since methyl bromide is highly volatile, nearly all environmental releases of this chemical are into the air. Thus, it is absorbed through inhalation, or through the skin, and eyes. When using any fumigant, fungicide, pesticide, or rodent killer, be sure to check the label, and if you see the presence of methyl bromide (and absolutely must use it), ensure adequate protective measures are taken.

■ Another form of bromide (potassium bromate), is used as a dough conditioner in some American commercial bakeries. In 1994 bromates were banned in Canada (for use in bread), however, in the U.S., only California has declared bromate to be a carcinogen. As a result, any bread product sold in California containing potassium bromate, has to display a cancer warning. This approach resulted in most California bakers ceasing to use potassium bromate. Since many national bakeries and fast food chains in the U.S. still use potassium bromate, it is wise to avoid baked goods that list "potassium bromate" or "bromated flour" among their ingredients. Potassium bromate is also used as an antiseptic, and astringent, in some mouthwash and toothpaste products.

■ Soft drinks (mostly the type containing citrus, such as Mountain Dew), and some energy drinks, are contaminated with brominated vegetable oil (BVO). BVO is used to suspend the flavoring throughout the beverage. This can be observed, as BVO creates a cloudy look to the beverage by evenly suspending the fruity flavor mixed into the drink—producing a look reminiscent of real fruit juice. It is only used where citrus ingredients are involved as they do not easily mix with water, and would normally separate—floating to the top, or sinking to the bottom of the beverage. This ingredient must be listed on the label, so look for it when purchasing such beverages.

■ Bromides are found in some medications—in the form of ipratropium bromide—primarily in nasal sprays, and inhalers, and in the form of methscopolamine bromide in some ulcer medications.

■ A type of bromide called benzalkonium is used in some cosmetics, and another form (sodium bromate) is found in some hair dyes, and permanent wave products.

- Sodium bromide is commonly found in hot tub sanitizers; those who want an alternative to bromide can use food-grade hydrogen peroxide.

- Brominated flame retardants are one of the most dangerous compounds found within modern vehicles, located in arm rests, door trim, and seats. When new cars heat up, they gas off these chemical compounds, causing us to inhale bromines. And, when fabrics with flame-retardants start to break down because of age, they release small particles of bromide-contaminated fibers that also are inhaled. Unfortunately, bromide is also commonly found in children's car safety seats. In a recent study, brominated flame-retardants were present in 44% of the children's car seats sampled.

- Our worst exposure to bromides is usually a result of its use as a fire-retardant (polybromo diphenyl ethers) on carpets, fabrics (especially pajamas for kids), mattresses, and upholstery. The real problem is these fabric-based products break down over time; the fire retardant becomes airborne (carried on small fibers), and we inhale it.

BROMIDE TOXICITY

Bromide builds up in the body, and aside from the damage it does as an endocrine disruptor, and iodine inhibitor, it also causes central nervous system problems. These problems can include psychiatric symptoms such as severe paranoia. In fact, as far back as the 1940's, psychiatry was aware bromide intoxication could result in mental conditions, ranging from depression to schizophrenia. (9)

One doctor found that, between 1920 and 1960, nearly a quarter of all hospital admissions for paranoid schizophrenia were due to bromide toxicity, caused by ingesting bromide-containing medications. In looking at emergency room visits prior to 1975—when bromine-containing sedatives were outlawed—it has been observed that bromine overdose resulted in diagnoses of brain damage, or psychosis. Such diagnoses resulted from bromide toxicity symptoms of depression, hallucinations, memory loss, seizures, and violent tendencies. Other symptoms of bromide toxicity include abdominal pain, acne, arrhythmia, fatigue, loss of appetite, rashes, skin lesions, and a metallic taste in the mouth.

Given its tendency to block iodine uptake, and to occupy those receptors, high bromide levels in the body are linked to thyroid conditions ranging from hypothyroidism to Hashimoto's disease (and other autoimmune thyroid conditions), and even thyroid cancer. One study found bromide levels were 50 times higher in thyroid cancer tissue than in normal thyroid tissue. (10)

In rat studies, brominated vegetable oil consumption caused heart and kidney damage (sometimes leading to kidney cancer), and resulted in fat deposits on these organs. Those rats also developed other symptoms, including testicular damage, stunted growth, and lethargy. In another rat study, kidney damage resulted from exposure to potassium bromate (in the form of a flame-retardant compound), along with permanent deafness. (11)

One physical symptom of bromide toxicity are "cherry angiomas", which are made up of clusters of capillaries on the surface of the skin. These take the form of small round domes, which may be flat-topped, ranging in color from bright red to purple. When they first develop, they may appear as small red dots the size of a pinpoint, but, over time, they can grow as large as a ¼ inch in diameter.

DETOXIFYING HALOGENS

According to Dr. Sircus (www.drsircus.com), the only effective way to remove bromides (and other halogens) from the body is to increase the intake of iodine. Iodine chelates (binds to) heavy metals and halogens, and carries them out of the body via urine.

This has the dual effect of detoxifying halogens out of the body, and decreasing their iodine inhibitory effects, by freeing up the blocked iodine receptors. (12)

When detoxifying bromides from the body many practitioners

suggest a salt loading protocol (based on the U.S. military's approach to bromide detoxification). The chloride in salt competes with bromide, so a person low in sodium chloride will hold more bromide, and conversely, high salt intake can greatly increase the excretion of bromide. Salt loading can also reduce side effects caused by bromide detoxification (including acne, anxiety, headache, fatigue, mouth and tongue sores, and twitching, jerking, or tingling sensations).

The salt loading protocol is as follows: drink ¼ - ½ teaspoon unrefined salt (such as Celtic or Himalayan), dissolved in ½ cup warm (purified or spring) water, followed immediately with 12-16 oz pure water. Repeat in 30-45 minutes if needed, and again, after a similar length of time, if symptoms persist. Iodine expert Dr. Brownstein suggests that one refrains from salt loading for more than a week.

If bromide detoxification symptoms do not decrease during that time, lower your dose of iodine for a while then work back up to the higher doses gradually. Salt loading is based on taking at least ½ tsp of salt daily, over and above one's regular usage. (For more details about the salt loading protocol, go to www.iodinehealth.wordpress.com/bromide-salt-loading.)

IODINE RESOURCES

For much more information on iodine, and its therapeutic use, visit the website www.iodineonmymind.com, and when there, be sure to click the link with the title "Drs. Brownstein, Abraham, and Flechas"—who operate out of the aforementioned Center for Holistic Medicine. This clinic uses very high levels of iodine to treat their patients, and these three doctors fully disagree with Dr. Gaby's findings (presented in the section on "Japanese Iodine Intake"). They have a full response to Dr. Gaby's position, which is well reasoned out, and based, in part, on many years of experience using high doses of iodine therapeutically.

This is an indication of their position on the issue: "We estimated the average daily intake of iodine by mainland Japanese in 1963 at

13.8 mg, based on information supplied by the Japanese Ministry of Health, which used only dry weight in their calculations, confirmed by a phone interview of one of us (GEA) on June 21, 2005."

Nonetheless, I have chosen to err on the side of caution, and thus recommend Dr. Gaby's approach (2 – 3 mg daily).

Endnotes

1. Venturi II, S., et al. "Role of iodine in evolution and carcinogenesis of thyroid, breast and stomach". Adv Clin Path. 4 (4): 11–17; 2000

2. Hollowell, J.G., et al. "Iodine Nutrition in the United States. Trends and Public Health Implications: Iodine Excretion Data from National Health and Nutrition Examination Surveys I and III (1971-1974 and 1988-1994)." J. of Clin. Endocr. & Metab., 83:3401-3408,1998

3. Dr. David Brownstein, Iodine, Why You Need It. Medical Alternative press, 2009

4. "Assessment of Japanese iodine intake based on seaweed consumption in Japan: A literature-based analysis." Theodore T Zava and David T Zava. Thyroid Research 2011, 4:14

5. Paediatric and Perinatal Epidemiology, 2012, 26, Suppl. 1, 108–117

6. The Lancet, Volume 382, Issue 9889, Pages 331 - 337, 27 July 2013

7. Group, Edward F.; 30 November 2012; "Iodine Deficiency and Autism linked in Research."

8. Can J Surg 1993;36:453-60

9. Levin M., "Transitory Schizophrenia Produced by Bromide Intoxication", Am J Psychiatry 1946

10. Malenchenko AF et al., "The Content and Distribution of Iodine, Chlorine and Bromide in the Normal and Pathologically Changed Thyroid Tissue." Med Radiol 1984

11. Morizono T et al., "The Effects of Cetrimide and Potassium Bromate on the Potassium Ion Concentration in the Inner Ear Fluid of the Guinea Pig." Physiol Bohemoslov 1988
12. Sticht, G., Käferstein, H., "Bromine. In Handbook on Toxicity of Inorganic Compounds." Seiler HG and Sigel, H Editors, Marcel Dekker Inc, 143-151, 1988

VITAMIN K2

In modern times, it is critical we consume sufficient amounts of vitamin K2—particularly because K2 deficiency has been clearly linked to two widespread ailments, osteoporosis, and heart disease (in the form of atherosclerosis, or calcification of the arteries). While these two serious conditions provide reason enough to supplement with vitamin K2, its benefits range far beyond simply protecting the arteries, and supporting skeletal structure. In fact, vitamin K2 also prevents and reverses a host of other modern ailments.

WHAT IS VITAMIN K?

In 1929, a Danish scientist discovered a compound eventually to be named vitamin K. Henrik Dam was studying the effects of cholesterol by feeding chickens a diet lacking in that fat. After a few weeks, he observed that the chickens fed only fat-depleted food developed hemorrhages, and started bleeding from tag sites (the place leg bands are attached). Furthermore, he found he could not reverse this by adding purified cholesterol back into their diet.

Soon, Dam realized there was an element in unpurified cholesterol, which prevented bleeding, and this he referred to as the "coagulation vitamin". This substance was later named vitamin K, simply because, in German, coagulation begins with a "K". From this discovery it was determined that serious vitamin K deficiencies would manifest as bleeding disorders, or malfunctions in blood clotting.

It is now known that vitamin K belongs to a family of vitamins that exist in various forms, including K1 (phylloquinone), K2 (menaquinone), and K3 (menadione). Both vitamins K1 and K2 activate certain coagulation factors, and are crucial for proper blood clotting. (However, there is no danger your coagulation factors will become overactive, if you take high amounts of vitamins K1, or K2.)

Vitamin K3 is a synthetic form, toxic in high doses, and, due to side effects, banned by the FDA from over-the-counter sales (although it may still be prescribed). Since it is of no value to us, vitamin K3 merits no further discussion at this time.

VITAMIN K1

Vitamin K1 (found in plant foods) is the most commonly available form of vitamin K in the modern diet. The foods richest in vitamin K1 include avocado, broccoli, Brussels sprouts, cabbage, cauliflower, kale, kiwi, grapes, parsley, spinach, and Swiss chard. While the absorption of K1 from green plants is usually low (cooked spinach is only 5% bio-available), absorption is improved by the addition of fat to the greens. With added fat, the bioavailability of K1 in spinach jumps to 13%.

Fat is responsible for this increased bioavailability because vitamin K is a fat-soluble vitamin, and—as with all fat-soluble vitamins—the presence of fat in the meal improves absorption. Therefore, oil-based salad dressings actually increase assimilation of fat-soluble nutrients in salads (not only vitamin K but also the carotenoids: beta-carotene, lutein, lycopene, and zeaxanthin).

In the famous "Framingham Study"—a long term, multi-generational study, begun in 1948 and still running today— lower risk for hip fracture was observed in those who consumed the most vitamin K1. However, another study attempted to get the same results with supplemental K1, and, in this form, vitamin K1 showed no benefits.

Therefore, K1 seems to have little value in supplemental form (at least for bone density), though it is clearly of value when obtained from the diet.

VITAMIN K2

Science has established that the type of vitamin K most utilized by the body is the K2 form. Vitamin K2 is found mostly in butter, egg yolks, and meat products—especially organ meats—from animals fed grass.

In North America, most food animals are fed grains as, it is cheap, and fattens animals up more than grass. Most cattle spend about 70% of their lives on pasture, and 30% eating grain-based rations (fattening them up before slaughter), while pigs, and poultry, eat grain-based diets throughout their lives.

This feeding of grain to industrial food animals has been the practice since about the 1930s. As a result, vitamin K2 deficiency has become widespread in the West, as has osteoporosis, and atherosclerosis.

Vitamin K2 is commonly found in the MK4 and MK7 forms, though K2 exists in other forms as well (MK5 through MK10). However, for our purposes, we will focus on MK4 and MK7, since they are the most researched, and can be purchased as supplements.

Vitamin K2, in the MK4 form, is found mostly in foods sourced from grass-fed animals. The MK7 form is created during fermentation, and is mostly found in certain cheeses, and in the fermented soybean food called natto. Unfortunately, this Japanese food is considered quite unpalatable to most North Americans, due to its "slimy" consistency, and intense smell and taste. Natto is the highest food source of vitamin K2 (1,100 mcg per 100 gr), with the next highest source being goose liver paté 369 mcg per 100 gr).

Even though some fermented foods contain K2, those with an appreciable amount are rare, since not every strain of bacteria can produce this vitamin. For example, yogurt contains very little, but

Brie and Gouda cheeses are relatively high in K2 (roughly 75 mcg per ounce).

Since K2 is produced by a specific strain of bacteria, these two cheeses do not require milk from grass-fed cows in order for there to be K2 present. However, if the milk does come from grass-fed cows, the K2 content will be even higher.

When shopping for dairy products, we often have to choose between grass-fed, and organic. My research indicates that certified organic dairy products must come from cows which have at least 30% of their diet derived from grasses. Thus, I will generally choose organic dairy products, since there will be some K2 present, and I do not have to worry about antibiotic or hormone residues.

WHY IS K2 SO IMPORTANT?

During growth vitamin K2 develops bones by directing calcium into the skeletal structure and cells. In adults, it works to maintain the health of bones and teeth.

The ability of K2 to maintain the skeletal structure in adults is demonstrated by its ability to keep bones healthy, and strong, in people experiencing bone loss from steroid use, dialysis, and/or paralysis.

When the body contains sufficient stores, vitamin K2 will continually direct calcium into bones and teeth, while keeping it away from the areas where it could do harm—such as the cardiovascular system. This is illustrated by a European study of more than 8,000 people (over the age of 55), which found that those with the highest intake of vitamin K2 had a 50% reduction in death by coronary heart disease. (1)

VASCULAR CALCIFICATION

The aforementioned study concluded vitamin K2 worked to reduce death from heart disease by preventing calcification ("hardening") of the arteries. This was confirmed by animal studies, which showed "MK-7 supplementation inhibited both vascular and myocardial calcification in CKD (Chronic Kidney Disease) animals on a high phosphate diet, and demonstrated a protective effect of MK-7 supplementation on early stages of cardiovascular calcification". (2) (Vitamin K1 was also tested but did not prevent arterial calcification.)

Furthermore, other animal studies have indicated arterial calcification may even be reversed with supplemental vitamin K2. (3) Therefore, those with hardening of the arteries would be well advised to take high amounts of vitamin K2, in order to reverse this disorder (along with lecithin, cayenne, garlic, pomegranate juice, and Omega 7 fatty acids).

Vascular calcification is now considered an independent risk factor for cardiovascular disease and mortality, especially in the elderly, and in patients with diabetes, and chronic kidney disease. In fact, calcification of the arteries is so counterproductive to cardiovascular health and longevity it is used as a measurement to predict biological age.

In one study, a group of over 10,000 people (in relatively good health), were followed for a period of five years, measuring their coronary artery calcium, and observing mortality from all causes. Ultimately there was found to be a direct relationship between their "observed age" (not their true, biological age), and the degree to which their arteries had calcified.

Those over 70 who had a low level of calcium in the arteries were considered to be 10 years younger (health-wise) than their peers. While those of a younger age, who had high amounts of calcium in their arteries, showed the equivalent of 30 years of extra age, over their true biological ages. (4)

In another study, showing the direct link between vitamin K2 and hardening of the arteries, 244 post-menopausal women took 180 mcg of a trademarked MK7 product, or a placebo, every day for three years. The researchers used ultrasound and pulse wave velocity to measure cardiovascular health, and arterial stiffness. By the end of the study, it was clear that the elasticity of the carotid artery had significantly improved in the group taking the vitamin K2, compared with the placebo group. "These results confirmed K2 not only inhibited age-related stiffening of the artery walls, but also made a statistically significant improvement in vascular elasticity." (5)

VITAMIN K2 DEFICIENCY

Up until recently, it was believed vitamin K deficiency only occurred if the intestinal tract was damaged, forbidding absorption of this nutrient. Since K2 (in the MK7 form) is produced mostly from K1 (by friendly bacteria in the gut), a deficiency was also often found among people who had been on broad-spectrum antibiotics, over long periods of time. In fact, heavy antibiotic use will reduce vitamin K2 production in the body by almost 75%.

In a manner similar to losing our ability to synthesize vitamin B12 in the intestines as we age, so too does vitamin K2 production get curtailed. Since much of the K2 in the body is converted from K1, a diet too low in the plant foods containing K1 will also reduce the amount of K2 in the body.

Even though we may eat plenty of plant foods, and be young enough to still convert K1 into K2 in our intestines, it appears the amount of the MK7 form created in the intestines may not be sufficient to meet the body's needs.

The MK4 version of K2 (unlike MK7) does not appear to be dependent on friendly bacteria, in order to be produced in the intestines. While it is also converted from K1, that conversion occurs in the arterial walls, pancreas, and testes. Yet, even in this case, we do not seem to produce enough of it to fulfill all of the body's requirements, and so some preformed K2 must be obtained from the diet and/or supplements.

SUPPLEMENTAL FORMS OF K2

Both the MK4 and MK7 version of K2 are available in supplemental form, though the effective dosages are very different. While K2 is not used medically for preventing osteoporosis in North America, in Japan health authorities have recommended it for this purpose since 1995. In fact, Japanese studies have indicated that MK4 can reduce fractures by up to 87%. (6)

The recommended dosage of MK4 required to treat osteoporosis is 45 mg daily, however, in Canada, the maximum amount of K2 allowed in a product is 120 mcg. Since MK4 is not effective in microgram doses, we in Canada can only use MK7, which, fortunately, is effective at these low doses.

The recommended amount of MK7, in the alternative health field, is about 120 mcg daily for maintenance, and twice that much for therapeutic use (though clinical studies often use 180 to 200 mcg). To put that into perspective, Japanese people who eat natto daily, ingest nearly 1,000 mcg of vitamin K2, in the MK7 form.

Certainly, there is much more science on the MK4 version of vitamin K2, but there are a few studies supporting MK7, and there are currently more studies underway. In at least one study, the MK7 form of K2 clearly showed effectiveness in stimulating bone formation, and inhibiting bone decline. (7)

Another MK7 study showed elevation in biomarkers of bone formation, along with inhibition of bone-reabsorbing factors found in parathyroid hormones. (8) As well, in 2011, the Singapore government approved a health supplement that contains the MK7 form of vitamin K2 (along with vitamin D3) for increasing bone density.

These data indicate that, while we Canadians do not have the choice as to which form of K2 we can purchase, we can at least take comfort in knowing that the form the government allows us to buy, has some scientific validity behind it.

VITAMIN K2 AND STROKE

The importance of vitamin K2 in preventing osteoporosis may be indicative of another valuable function it also performs. In a "Study of Osteoporotic Fractures", it was shown bone density is a good general predictor of mortality. This study found every standard deviation from normal bone density led to a 20% greater risk of mortality in older women. An update to this study further confirmed the findings of the original study. It concluded a 1.23 times greater risk of dying, if a subject had one or more back fractures, and severe osteoporosis increased the risk of dying from a lung-related disorder by 2.6 times. (9)

What the study update discovered was the women with osteoporosis did not die from complications from broken bones, or the resulting surgery—falling accounted for only about 3% of the mortalities. The majority of deaths occurred mostly from cancer, heart attack, and stroke. These kinds of studies indicate osteoporosis is a warning sign that calcium has built up in the arteries, instead of remaining in the bones where it belongs. This material clearly ties into the study referred to previously (under "Vascular Calcification"), in which subjects had their coronary artery calcium measured, and vascular calcification was linked to increased "mortality from all causes".

Now, the underlying cause of stroke is pretty much the same as the cause of a heart attack: damaged blood vessels. Until recently, the belief was a high sodium diet caused hypertension and strokes. However, not long ago, The Journal of the American Medical Association concluded that, "… results do not support a general recommendation to reduce sodium intake".

Recent studies have shown another mineral affecting blood pressure (calcium), may be more likely than sodium to cause hypertension. The repeated link between high calcium intake (1200–1500 mg supplemental), and stroke and heart disease, supports the concept that calcium build-up in the arteries is logically linked to causing strokes. (This material is covered in more detail in Health Secrets: Volume One.)

In the aforementioned "Study of Osteoporotic Fractures", one standard deviation from the norm of bone density was equal to a three times increased risk of having a stroke, and a 1.7 times increased risk for hypertension. Further supporting this theory are studies showing diets high in vitamin K prevent thickening of the arteries, in a species of rat bred to be stroke-prone.

INFLAMMATION AND VITAMIN K2

It well known inflammation is the root cause of many ailments, including cancer, heart disease, diabetes, and arthritis. The older we get, the more we produce the inflammatory compound Interleukin-6—a chemical messenger known as a cytokine, which is part of our immune system. When produced in normal amounts, it is a necessary component of a healthy immune system, but when it overwhelms the other cytokines, IL-6 causes excessive inflammation.

Findings from the National Research Institute in Italy, confirm this by showing IL-6 to be concentrated in damaged blood vessels and arthritic joints. Their study revealed people with the highest amount of IL-6 were nearly twice as likely to develop mobility-related ailments.

Elevated levels of IL-6 are also found in people with symptoms of Alzheimer's disease, another disease characterized by symptoms of inflammation. (10) Fortunately, vitamin K2 inhibits both the overproduction of IL-6, and general inflammation.

ALZHEIMER'S DISEASE AND VITAMIN K2

Some years ago, a research scientist at the University of North Carolina discovered hemodialysis patients were more prone to bone fractures. At the same time, they had higher than normal levels of a compound called "apolipoprotein E" in their blood. The scientist (Dr. M. Kohlmeier) suspected these people might also be prone to poor vitamin K status, or may not absorb or produce it well. Eventually studies confirmed this fact, and elevated levels of this apoE compound were later also directly linked to Alzheimer's disease.

The combination of low vitamin K, along with high apoE, affects the body's ability to regulate calcium levels in the brain. And indeed, studies have found patients with Alzheimer's disease have unhealthy calcium levels in their brains.

K2 AND INSULIN REGULATION

The fact that some of the highest levels of stored vitamin K2 are in the pancreas, has led to the idea it may also be a necessary part of controlling blood sugar levels. Japanese scientists studied the link between vitamin K, and insulin function in the body, and (though it was an animal study) what occurred with vitamin K deficiency mimicked what occurs with diabetes. The deficiency in vitamin K interfered with clearance of glucose from the blood, and then stimulated an excessive insulin release. (11)

There was a small-scale human study, performed in 2011, which concluded, "To summarize, we have demonstrated for the first time that vitamin K2 supplementation for 4 weeks increased insulin sensitivity in healthy young men". (12)

Considering insulin malfunction is linked not only to diabetes, but also to the risk of developing certain types of cancer and Alzheimer's disease, the importance of taking adequate amounts of vitamin K2 proves even more obvious.

AUTISM

Vitamin K2 deficiency causes calcium to be unregulated in the body, allowing it to deposit, and form calcium oxalate crystals. This mechanism led researcher Catherine Tamaro, B.S.M.E., to propose vitamin K2 deficiency may cause many of the symptoms associated with autism. Her premise is supported by studies showing calcium oxalate crystals are found in many autistic children (often in the form of kidney stones).

Since one of the functions of calcium is to trigger firing of neurons in the brain, an excess of calcium in the blood can cause the neurons to over-fire, until they actually die. Tamaro therefore suggests the addition of vitamin K2 to the diet of those with autism would activate bone proteins that regulate calcium. This would reduce over-firing of these neurotransmitters, while aiding in calming the brain.

Vitamin K2 deficiency can also cause chronic neuronal hyper-excitement, which would manifest in the form of some autism-like symptoms in those who are not technically "autistic".

Certain substances, known as "excitotoxins", also trigger hyper-excitement in the brain. Excitotoxins include aspartame, glutamic acid, and MSG, all linked to autism, and other neurological disorders. These excitotoxins also cause an imbalance in calcium regulation, which leads to inflammation, and ultimately to the death of neurons.

K2 AND CANCER

Now a look at studies linking vitamin K2 deficiency to increased cancer risk.

The "European Prospective Investigation into Cancer and Nutrition" involved over 24,000 participants, from the ages of 35 to 64—all of whom were free of cancer when enrolled in the study. The participants were tracked for an average of 10 years, and part of the study looked at their vitamin K1 and K2 dietary intake over these years, comparing it to cancer incidence and mortality. The study revealed vitamin K2 (but not K1) status was inversely associated with the risk of developing, and dying from, cancer.

The researchers concluded, the "intake of menaquinones, which is highly determined by the consumption of cheese, is associated with a reduced risk of incident and fatal cancer". (Certain types of cheeses—specifically Brie, Edam, and Gouda—represent the few appreciable sources of vitamin K2 found in the modern Western diet.)

The benefits of vitamin K2 intake was (for unknown reasons) better for men than women, especially showing a dramatic reduction in both lung and prostate cancers.

Observations from this study indicated the higher the intake of K2, the lower the risk of all forms of prostate cancer. However, the most significant protection offered by vitamin K2 was against advanced prostate cancer, where it was associated with a 63% reduction in risk. (13) If you are a man, this alone is reason enough to start supplementing with vitamin K2.

At the Mayo Clinic in Minnesota, researchers have found people who have higher intakes of vitamin K have a lower risk of developing non-Hodgkin lymphoma. And, in this study, even vitamin K1 showed a preventative value in reducing cancer risk. Those who had the highest levels of vitamin K1, from diet and/or supplements, had a 45% less risk for developing this form of lymphoma. (14)

Meanwhile, in Japan, researchers discovered vitamin K2 may play a role in preventing the type of liver cancer caused by viral cirrhosis. In a 2004 study, involving 40 women with viral liver cirrhosis, half the women received 45 mg vitamin K2 per day (in the MK4 form of K2). The participants were followed for just over 7 years, after which it was determined vitamin K2 supplementation decreased the risk of the development of liver cancer in these subjects—though possibly by just delaying the onset of cancer.

The researchers believe that a by-product of vitamin K2 (geranyl-geraniol) induced cell death in tumor cells, preventing proliferation of cancer cells. The researchers wrote, "The study indicates that vitamin K2 decreases the risk of liver cancer to about 20% compared to the control group". (15)

ANTIOXIDANT PROPERTIES OF K2

Free radical damage in the body—caused by toxins, radiation, and reactive oxygen molecules—are a cause of cancer, heart disease, inflammatory conditions, and premature aging. Since vitamin K2 serves as an antioxidant as well (over and above its many other functions), it is also an important part of our body's basic survival mechanisms.

One study subjected test animals to extreme free radical damage, finding that vitamin K2 alone protected their livers from induced oxidative stress. Another study showed vitamin K2 to be almost as effective as vitamin E in preventing oxidation of fatty acids—a benchmark of its antioxidant activity. (16)

BLOOD THINNING DRUGS AND K2

If we see a link between vitamin K deficiency and increased cancer rates, then we have to wonder what effect blood-thinning drugs will have on cancer.

Since some of these drugs (Warfarin and Coumadin) work by blocking vitamin K from doing its blood-clotting function, patients are advised not to eat foods, or supplements, containing vitamin K (1 or 2). (Some of the newer blood thinning drugs, such as dabigatran (Pradaxa) and rivaroxaban (Xarelto) do not block vitamin K—but nonetheless still have dangerous side effects, and should be avoided if possible.)

Given that blood-thinning drugs, which disable vitamin K activity, also impede its antioxidant functions, they must expose cells to higher amounts of free radical damage. The type of damage that can lead to cancer growth.

Indeed, a recent study looked for just that link, examining Warfarin use in men who had developed prostate cancer. There appeared to be no danger for the first 2 years of using Warfarin, but for those taking Warfarin for 4 or more years, there was a 220% increased risk of developing advanced prostate cancer. According to the authors of this study, this finding can be explained as simply being the result of long-term depletion of antioxidant activity in the body, caused by blocking vitamin K uptake. (17)

K2 AND PARKINSON'S DISEASE

Recent research on vitamin K2, published in the journal Science, has given new hope to people with Parkinson's disease. Neuroscientist, Patrik Verstreken, stated, "It appears from our research that administering vitamin K2 could possibly help patients with Parkinson's. However, more work needs to be done to understand this better".

In people who have Parkinson's, mitochondrial activity is dysfunctional, resulting in mitochondria no longer producing sufficient energy for the cell.

The mitochondria are like power plants, which drive the operation of each cell. They are found in every cell of the body (except red blood cells), and convert the energy of food molecules into ATP, which powers most cell functions.

As the cells in parts of the brain start dying off, communication between neurons is disrupted, resulting in the symptoms of Parkinson's (lack of movement, tremors, and muscle stiffness).

Several genetic defects have been found in Parkinson's patients, two of which both lead to reduced mitochondrial activity. By studying these genetic mutations, scientists hope to get closer to understanding the mechanisms underlying Parkinson's disease.

The research referred to at the beginning of this section, involved giving vitamin K2 to experimental fruit flies, who had defective mitochondria (as with Parkinson's patients). The flies with the genetic defect, akin to the one associated with Parkinson's, had lost their ability to fly, but, once they were supplemented with K2, their ability to fly was restored.

It was determined that energy production was restored due to the effect vitamin K2 had on improving electron transport within the mitochondria. This also implies benefit for conditions like chronic fatigue syndrome, and fibromyalgia, or any condition where physical energy levels are dangerously low.

Vitamin D is also required for healthy function of the mitochondria. Researchers from Newcastle University found that muscle function improved with vitamin D supplementation. The lead author of the study (Dr Akash Sinha) said, "We have proved for the first time a link between vitamin D and mitochondria function".

DENTAL HEALTH AND K2

We know vitamin K2 helps to maintain the teeth, as well as the rest of the skeletal system. However, the importance of K2 for dental health is emphasized by the knowledge that, after the pancreas, the highest amount of K2 stored in tissues is found in the salivary glands. In fact, even if rats are fed only vitamin K1, almost all of the vitamin K found in their salivary glands will exist in the form of K2. (18)

Believe it or not, as far back as 1945, science was aware of the value of vitamin K in preventing cavities. American researchers conducted a proper double blind, placebo-controlled study of chewing gum that contained a precursor to vitamin K2 (menadione). Chewing the gum reduced incidence of new cavities, and caused a dramatic drop in L. acidophilus, the bad bacteria in the mouth linked to causing cavities. (L. acidophilus is a beneficial bacteria when it resides in the gut, but not so in the mouth.)

An attempt to repeat this study failed to produce the same results, and research was abandoned. At the time, it was assumed the menadione (technically vitamin K3) had worked because it was antibacterial. However, this is unlikely, since the concentration of menadione in the mouth would not have been sustained long enough to kill appreciable amounts of bad bacteria.

A decade later, German researchers tried injecting menadione into the abdominal cavities of hamsters. They found this approach to be more effective at preventing tooth decay, than adding the K3 to their food. Even though these studies indicated more research on the subject of vitamin K and cavities was warranted, no further research on the subject was pursued. It is a shame they did not try using K2, instead of K3, but drug companies are well aware one cannot patent a natural vitamin—though you can patent a synthetic variation (such as K3).

Now, as we gain greater understanding of the role of vitamin K in the body, it is becoming obvious that the K2 form of vitamin K is necessary for good dental health.

DR. WESTON A. PRICE AND DENTAL HEALTH

In the 1930s and 40s, dentist Dr. Weston A. Price (1870-1948) was motivated to search for reasons why Americans had such poor dental health. Dr. Price traveled the world to study humans who had not modernized, and were still following their ancient, traditional diets. These included communities in the Outer Hebrides, Inuit, Polynesian Islanders, African tribes, Australian Aborigines, New Zealand Maori, and the indigenous peoples of North and South America. In all these areas, he found the inhabitants to have mostly perfect teeth and dental arches, almost no tooth decay, and superior general health and resistance to disease.

His research ultimately concluded that a traditional diet high in vitamins A, D, and K, together, could not only prevent cavities but could also work to reverse them. (For more information on his amazing research, go to www.westonaprice.org.) As a result, Price suggested the best foods for preventing, and reversing, dental cavities were cod liver oil and grass-fed butter oil—natural sources of vitamins A, D, and K2. In fact, he would often put his clients on this regimen instead of drilling and filling cavities.

There are three calcified tissues which form teeth—the cementum forms the roots, the enamel forms the surface, and the dentin forms the support structure beneath the enamel. Cells called odontoblasts line the surface of the pulp just below the dentin, and continually produce new dentin material. If a cavity invades the dentin and infects these cells, they can die. However, pulp tissue contains stem cells that can differentiate into new odontoblasts, and, if the right nutrients are present, this has the ability to regenerate damaged dentin. (19)

We now know the growth and re-mineralization of the dentin, which Dr. Price observed as a response to feeding his patients cod liver oil, and grass-fed butter oil, was a result of providing the dentin its 3 essential co-factors—vitamins A, D, and K2. (Price referred to K2 as "Activator X", since K2 had yet to be "discovered".)

Dentin produces osteocalcin (a protein that requires vitamin K), which channels calcium into the skeletal system. Since dentin creates more osteocalcin than bone does, we know that osteocalcin plays an important role in the growth of new dentin. This production of osteocalcin is also dependent on vitamins A and D.

THE ROLE OF VITAMIN A

Those familiar with my other writings know I believe vitamin A deficiency to be widespread, and that the dangers of too much vitamin A has been overplayed in the media. Dr. Price found that a traditional diet contained as much as 10 times more vitamin A than the standard Western diet of his time period—today we eat even less foods containing vitamin A.

Vitamins A and D are necessary (along with vitamin K2) in order for the body to produce osteocalcin, and MGP (matrix gla protein). Both these substances are required for moving calcium around the body, and ensuring it arrives at the proper location. Without vitamins A and D, these protein substances cannot be made, but without vitamin K2 they cannot be activated. Therefore, when supplementing with one of them, we should ensure we have adequate amounts of the other two.

Many people are supplementing with high levels of vitamin D, but are forgetting about vitamin A, a co-factor of vitamin D. In nature both nutrients are found together in the primary food source (fish or mammal livers), and would normally be consumed together. Now that we are taking nutrients in isolated forms (supplements), it becomes more of a balancing act.

It is most likely that the potential toxicity of excessive vitamin A may be due to the ensuing deficiency of vitamin D that follows—and vice versa. Fat-soluble nutrients are so interdependent that taking one fat-soluble vitamin creates a need for the others. I have repeatedly found studies showing the dangers of supplementing with high levels of vitamins A, or D, are based on taking them in isolation, and not in tandem.

Vitamin A is necessary for development and maintenance of the skeletal system because it is required for the production and activity of osteoclast cells, which break down old bone material. This process is necessary to recycle bone tissue, both for maintaining bone density, and for repairing fractured or broken bones.

Vitamin D produces osteoblasts, those cells that build up bone structure. So, after vitamin A breaks down old bone material, vitamin D steps in to help with rebuilding new bone tissue. Now, vitamin D can produce osteoblasts on its own, but when there is adequate vitamin A present, a synergistic effect occurs which produces more osteoblasts than vitamin D can make alone.

Some have stated vitamin A is dangerous because it can cause osteoporosis, due to this production of osteoclasts. However, they are overlooking the fact that, when vitamin D is present in adequate amounts, the next step occurs—the broken-down bone material is then used to build up new bone compounds. Thus, vitamin A and D are complementary, and are both are required for good bone and teeth health.

One major point in favor of vitamin A is it has a vitamin K2-sparing action. Therefore, when we have good stores of vitamin A in the body, there is less of a need for K2. Unfortunately, if one takes high doses of vitamin A as a supplement, without adequate vitamin

D, eventually it can lead to osteoporosis, in part due to the reduced levels of vitamin K2. And, if we take high levels of vitamin D without K2, the body will mobilize too much calcium into the bloodstream—leading to hypercalcemia.

As discussed at the beginning, K2 is essential to preventing vascular calcification since part of the function of vitamin K2 in regulating calcium in the body is to remove calcium from arterial plaque. After it has done that, it is vitamin A which then removes the unwanted calcium from the body.

Recommended amounts of vitamin A and D vary depending on whom you talk to, but one thing is evident—as long as you have a reasonable amount of each, you will not have to worry about toxic overload from any excess of the other.

VITAMIN K2 AND D3

Combining vitamin D3 with K2 is more effective at building bones than either one used alone. (20) The combination is necessary because, while vitamin D helps us to absorb the calcium, the vitamin K directs it into the skeletal structure.

Science has long known vitamin D is essential for the absorption of calcium, but now we know it is the vitamin K2 that directs the calcium into the skeleton—while preventing it from being deposited in the organs, joints, and arteries.

There is now evidence the safety of vitamin D3 is dependent on one's vitamin K2 status. In fact, vitamin D toxicity may be a result of vitamin K2 deficiency (as well as the aforementioned vitamin A deficiency). So vitamin D3 mobilizes calcium into the bloodstream, but if K2 is not present to channel the calcium into the bones, the calcium may build up plaque on the arterial walls—leading to atherosclerosis.

Vitamins K2 and D3 work together to increase matrix Gla protein. This protein is responsible for protecting your blood vessels from calcification, and preventing hardening of the arteries. MGP status is so important that it can be used as a laboratory measure of your vascular and cardiac status (if you have a doctor progressive enough to give you such a test).

The body stores most of the vitamin D it obtains from sunshine in an inactive form—converting it into an active form, as required. Therefore, we should be careful with vitamin D supplements, as they are the active form of D3. In other words, we are ingesting an "end product" instead of a precursor. Precursors are building blocks, which allow the body to produce as much of the end product as it optimally requires. Thus, anyone taking more than 5,000 IU of vitamin D3 daily should definitely add a vitamin K2 supplement to their regimen, for that reason alone.

OTHER POSSIBLE BENEFITS OF VITAMIN K2

Ongoing research into the properties of vitamin K2 reveal more areas of benefit.

One intriguing discovery is the preferential retention of vitamin K2 found in the testes of male rats. This, when considered in conjunction with the fact human sperm contains a vitamin K dependent protein, implies it is necessary for healthy fertility.

Another recent finding is the kidneys store large amounts of vitamin K2. The kidneys also secrete a protein component dependent on K2—one that prevents the formation of calcium salts. We now know those who have kidney stones only secrete this protein component in an inactive form—a form which poorly inhibits the development of kidney stones. This suggests K2 may be an important piece of the puzzle as to why some people develop kidney stones more often than others do. (21)

Since vitamin K2 can remove accumulated calcification and plaque from veins and arteries (according to rat studies, and one human trial), it may also help prevent the formation of varicose veins. And, with regular supplementation, may even work to reverse this condition.

Vitamin K2 may also prevent the wrinkling of skin. This idea is based on studies that show women with low bone density tend toward deep facial wrinkles, and those with better bone density show less of a predisposition to skin wrinkles. As well, research published in 2008 (in the journal Nephrology), showed wrinkling of the face to be associated with reduced kidney function—which is linked to vitamin K2 deficiency. Since it is known Japanese women show less skin wrinkling than North Americans, and they have one of the few diets in the world still high in K2 (due to eating natto), it seems evident that K2 status will show on our faces as well as in our bones.

WHAT DEPLETES VITAMIN K2?

Excessive antibiotic use can kill off intestinal flora, thereby negatively affecting the ability of the body to create vitamin K2 from K1 found in the diet.

Any substances that interfere with absorbing fat-soluble nutrients can reduce vitamin K levels. This includes drugs that reduce cholesterol, Olestra (fat substitute), fat-blocking supplements, and even low fat diets. In the case of low fat diets, remember the oil found in salad dressing allows the vitamin K1 in leafy greens to be properly absorbed.

Mineral oil, commonly used as a laxative, can prevent absorption of vitamin K, and the preservative BHT interferes with the function of vitamin K.

Vitamin K deficiency can also be caused by gallstones, diseases of the GI tract, liver disease, lack of a gallbladder, and estrogen drugs.

WARNINGS

There is no known toxicity associated with high doses of vitamin K2 in the forms of MK4 or MK7. While the body uses vitamin K2 for purposes of blood clotting, studies have indicated high doses of MK4 (135 mg daily, divided dose), showed no risk of abnormal blood clotting.

As for MK7—used in microgram doses rather than milligrams—
one usually takes 120 mcg daily (the legal limit in Canada). However,
for osteoporosis, or atherosclerosis, one should take at least 240 mcg
per day, perhaps more. Since the intake of MK7 among Japanese
people who eat natto is about 1,000 mcg daily, there are no worries
about overdosing with MK7 either.

Vitamin K2 is generally safe to take during pregnancy and lacta-
tion, and should be, since K2 deficiency can cause birth defects.

Extremely high levels of supplemental vitamin E (above 1200 IU
daily) can affect vitamin K's ability to coagulate blood, if vitamin K
levels are dangerously low in the body.

People on blood thinning drugs, such as Warfarin, Coumadin or
Heparin, should not take vitamin K, since these drugs work by interfering with vitamin K activity in the body. People on these drugs are
advised not to eat too many greens, due to the vitamin K1 content
of these foods. That means those on such drugs are going to be seriously deficient in vitamin K. And, in fact, studies do show those on
anticoagulants for long periods tend towards having osteoporosis,
atherosclerosis, and higher risks of stroke, than average.

Since vitamin K is a fat-soluble nutrient, if you are taking it in a
softgel pill form (more effective than powder or tablets), you need to
take it at a meal containing fat, in order to fully absorb it. This does
not hold true with liquid vitamin K2 products, which can be taken
under the tongue, and will absorb through the mouth. Liquid vitamin K2 products are of special value to those trying to protect their
teeth naturally, since the K2 goes to work in the mouth immediately.

Endnotes

1. Geleijnse J.M., et al, "Dietary intake of menaquinone is associated with a reduced risk of coronary heart disease, The Rotterdam study," Journal of Nutrition, 143 (11): Nov; 2004

2. Scheiber D et al. "High-dose menaquinone-7 supplementation reduces cardiovascular calcification in a murine model of extraosseous calcification." Nutrients. 2015, 7

3. Blood. 2007 Apr 1; 109(7):2823-31, "Regression of warfarin-induced medial elastocalcinosis by high intake of vitamin K in rats." Schurgers LJ, et al.

4. Shaw LJ, et al. "Coronary artery calcium as a measure of biologic age."Atherosclerosis. 2006; 188(1):112-119

5. Knapen MHJ et al. "Menaquinone-7 Supplementation Improves Arterial Stiffness In Healthy Postmenopausal Women: Double-Blind Randomised Clinical Trial." Thrombosis Haemostasis. 2015; 19(5):113

6. Sato, Y; Kanoko T, Satoh K, Iwamoto J (2005). "Menatetrenone and vitamin D2 with calcium supplements prevent nonvertebral fracture in elderly women with Alzheimer's disease". Bone 36 (1): 61–8.

7. Yamaguchi M, November 2006. "Regulatory mechanism of food factors in bone metabolism and prevention of osteoporosis." Yakugaku Zasshi 126 (11): 1117–37

8. Tsukamoto Y (2004). "Studies on action of menaquinone-7 in regulation of bone metabolism and its preventive role of osteoporosis". BioFactors 22 (1-4): 5–19

9. Browner WS, et al. 1991. "Non-trauma mortality in elderly women with low bone mineral density." Study of Osteoporotic Fractures Research Group. Lancet 338:355-58.

10. Ferrucci L, et al. 1999. "Serum IL-6 level and the development of disability in older persons." J Am Geriatr Soc 47:639-46.

11. Sakamoto N, et al. 1999. "Low vitamin K intake effects on glucose tolerance in rats." Int J Vit Nutr Res 69:27-31

12. Hyung Jin Choi, MD, et al. "Vitamin K2 Supplementation Improves Insulin Sensitivity via Osteocalcin Metabolism: A Placebo-Controlled Trial." Diabetes Care September 2011 vol. 34 no. 9 e147

13. Am J Clin Nutr. 2010, May; 91(5). "Dietary vitamin K intake in relation to cancer incidence and mortality: results from the Heidelberg cohort of the European Prospective Investigation into Cancer and Nutrition (EPIC-Heidelberg)". Nimptsch K, et al.

14. Mayo Clinic. "Vitamin K may protect against developing non-Hodgkin's lymphoma, say Mayo Clinic researchers." ScienceDaily, 21 April 2010

15. Habu D, et al. "Role of vitamin K2 in the development of hepatocellular carcinoma in women with viral cirrhosis of the liver." JAMA, 2004 Jul 21; 292(3):358-61

16. Vervoort LM, et al. 1997. "The potent antioxidant activity of the vitamin K cycle in microsomal lipid peroxidation." Biochem Pharmacol 54:871-6

17. Tagalakis V, Tamim H. "The effect of warfarin use on clinical stage and histological grade of prostate cancer." Pharmacoepidemiol Drug Saf. 2010 May 19(5):436-9

18. Zacharski LR, Rosenstein R. "Reduction of Salivary Tissue Factor (Thromboplastin) Activity by Warfarin Therapy." Blood. 1979; 53(3): 366-374

19. Huang GT-J, et al. "Formation of Odontoblast-Like Cells from Cultured Human Dental Pulp Cells on Dentin In Vitro." J Endod. 2006; 32: 1066-1073

20. Weber P., "Vitamin K and Bone Health," Nutrition, 17: 880-887; 2001

21. Vermeer C, et al. "Vitamin K and the Urogenital Tract." Haemostasis. 1986; 16: 246-257

MAGNESIUM

One of the most common nutritional deficiencies today is that of the essential mineral magnesium. As with many other nutrients, this deficiency is due to the over-processing of foods, topsoil erosion, and modern farming techniques, which leave soil (and the crops grown in it) starved for minerals.

However, in the case of magnesium, the problem is compounded by the fact most people consume dairy products high in calcium. High calcium intake, in effect, steals magnesium from the body, and most people do not eat enough unprocessed whole foods to offset that dietary imbalance. As well, magnesium is one mineral the body uses high amounts of—especially in times of stress—and it does not store as well as most other minerals. Therefore, in most cases, we need to supplement with magnesium, and not rely exclusively on diet to provide enough to keep us in optimal health.

WHY IS MAGNESIUM SO IMPORTANT?

The critical importance of magnesium is indicated by the fact that magnesium ions are necessary for all living cells, and over 300 enzymes in the body require magnesium ions to function. As well, magnesium is necessary for the production of adenosine triphosphate

(ATP) for cellular energy, and DNA and RNA, required for healthy cell turnover and reducing the effects of aging.

Of the hundreds of biochemical reactions magnesium is involved in, three are critical to our good health. Magnesium is as important as calcium to keep the bones strong; it is necessary to maintain a proper heart rhythm; and it keeps the nervous system functioning efficiently.

Our body stores around half of its magnesium inside cells found in the organs and tissues. The majority of the remaining magnesium is combined with calcium and phosphorus, and is stored in the bones. And, about one percent of magnesium in the body circulates at a constant level, within the blood.

The importance of magnesium was emphasized to me a few years ago upon reading an editorial in Life Extension Magazine. The editor stated if we were to fortify our drinking water with magnesium—so people received roughly 200 mg of extra magnesium daily—we would cut heart disease rates in half. Being aware heart disease is the leading cause of death in the Western world, that revelation had a big impact on me.

Supporting this thesis is the World Health Organization, which has recommended drinking water should ideally contain from 25 to 50 mg of magnesium per liter—an amount which would dramatically reduce deaths from heart attack, and stroke. Here in North America, most bottled water averages less than 5 mg of magnesium per liter, while bottled water in the other parts of the world averages about 20 mg of magnesium per liter. However, low levels of magnesium in our drinking water is only one reason why magnesium deficiency is common throughout North America.

MAGNESIUM DEFICIENCY

Here is a shocking statistic: according to a clinical study published in The Journal of Intensive Care Medicine, if you are deficient in magnesium you are twice as likely to die as someone who is not deficient. (1)

Nearly 50% of Americans are considered magnesium deficient, which we can easily extrapolate to Canadians as well. (2) In fact, research published in the American Journal of Epidemiology (2002) revealed that, when the diets of over 2,500 children (ages 11-19) were analyzed, fewer than 14% of boys, and 12% of girls, had an adequate intake of magnesium.

As with most severe nutritional deficiencies, that of magnesium is widespread due to modern living. One reason is the excessive consumption of dairy products (high in calcium), combined with a lack of unprocessed organic grains, nuts and vegetables (high in magnesium). Since too much calcium will deplete the body of magnesium, this dietary imbalance is a strong contributing factor. Another modern dietary cause of magnesium deficiency is high sugar intake, which also depletes the body of magnesium.

Then we have modern food processing techniques—especially the refining of grains—which removes most of the magnesium found in these staple foods. As well, non-organic farming practices deplete the soil of magnesium, and other minerals, and, by extension, the foods grown in such soil. When topsoil has eroded, and the fertilizers used are synthetic, and limited to three minerals (nitrogen, phosphorous and potassium), magnesium is not available to be taken up into the plants. Therefore, magnesium is not present in those foods—yet another reason to purchase organic foods as often as possible.

As well, taking certain medications (including antacids) disrupt magnesium absorption, while other medications (like diuretics and insulin) cause the body to excrete higher than normal amounts of magnesium.

MAGNESIUM VS CALCIUM

Most of you will be familiar with the 2 to 1 ratio of calcium to magnesium found in supplements, as that is the traditional ratio recommended. What this essentially means is that every 500 mg of calcium ingested will need, or use up, 250 mg of magnesium. Since our diet tends to be higher in calcium than magnesium—especially if we use dairy products on a daily basis—and since calcium will essentially rob the body of what little magnesium is present, dairy food consumption can contribute to magnesium deficiency. This will not occur if one consumes little or no dairy products, and eats many whole plant foods.

Another reason magnesium deficiency is widespread is outdated advice from doctors, suggesting women take 1000 to 1500 mg of calcium daily. This is often on top of the calcium they receive from their diet (which is already high, if their diet includes dairy products). Recommending this amount of calcium is overkill, illustrated by the fact average intake of calcium from a traditional diet does not generally exceed 500 mg daily, and is usually closer to 300 mg.

Furthermore, cultures that ingested low amounts of calcium from their traditional diets (since they did not consume dairy products), showed very low incidence of osteoporosis. (These include African, Chinese, and Japanese, cultures.) However, since the diet of these groups has now become more akin to the Western diet, their problems with osteoporosis are now on the increase.

For all the medical emphasis on calcium being necessary for preventing osteoporosis, at least two clinical studies found inadequate magnesium intake lowered bone density. Whereas, sufficient magnesium intake (even only through dietary sources) increased bone density—thereby reducing the risk of osteoporosis, and bone fractures. "In both studies, we found that the higher the intake [of magnesium], the higher the level of bone mineral density," said K. L. Tucker, PhD, professor at the Friedman School of Nutrition Science and Policy at Tufts University. "This is no surprise, since magnesium is needed for the body to properly utilize calcium and vitamin D, both of which are necessary for strong bones." (3)

Even worse, in the past few years, more than one study has linked calcium supplements to heart disease and strokes, in postmenopausal women. Those studies did not go so far as to make the link between excessive calcium and correspondingly low levels of magnesium, but at least now the dialogue should begin in the scientific community. (This subject has been covered in more detail, in Health Secrets: Volume One.)

MAGNESIUM DEFICIENCY SYMPTOMS

The simple way I describe the function of magnesium to those I consult with is to clench my fist and say, "this is what calcium does," and then open my hand and say, "this is what magnesium does". It is more complex than that, of course, but basically, calcium is the contractor, and magnesium the relaxer, and as a relaxer, magnesium also dilates. So, too much calcium, and/or not enough magnesium, leads to over-contracted muscles and/or constricted blood vessels.

Thus, the most common magnesium deficiency symptoms include cramping, or spasms, in the legs or feet (especially at night), headaches, and, more dangerously, irregular heartbeat, and high blood pressure. Here, the headaches—and sometimes migraines as well—and the hypertension, are due to blood flow being inhibited by constricted blood vessels, and are relieved by the vasodilation magnesium allows. I have often seen such symptoms clear up, within a week to a month, after recommending a high quality magnesium supplement, taken at a therapeutic dose level.

Because this nutrient is critical to our health, when we lack magnesium, we are open to damage from environmental contaminants, heavy metals, and radiation. Without adequate magnesium, the body accumulates toxins, becomes acidic, begins to degenerate, and ages prematurely.

Initially, a magnesium deficiency interferes with nerve and

muscle impulses, so a slight magnesium deficiency will first show up symptomatically as mild depression, and a general lack of well-being. As the deficiency worsens headaches, lower back pain, and stiff muscles—particularly in the back, neck, and shoulders—follow. If the deficiency continues for too long, symptoms will include calcium deposits, hypertension, muscle cramps, muscle spasms, and twitches.

At this point, one starts to feel constantly fatigued, and sleeping will become difficult, and not particularly restful. Finally, when symptoms become severe, one experiences body spasms, and/or involuntary and abnormal muscular contractions and jerks; the heart can start racing and can go out of rhythm (arrhythmia), leading to angina pectoris (serious heart pains).

Long-term magnesium deficiency can lead to calcium deficiency, alcoholic hallucinations (excess alcohol depletes magnesium), unusual face and eye movement, alopecia (baldness), swollen gums, and lesions of the gums. When magnesium deficiency affects the brain and nervous system, symptoms may include anxiety, Attention Deficit Disorder, confusion, depression, disorientation, hyperactivity, irritability, lack of coordination, and personality changes.

While not exclusive to magnesium deficiency, these other physical symptoms can also occur: asthma, bone spurs, chronic fatigue, colon cancer, fibromyalgia, gastrointestinal disorders, IBS, irritable bladder, kidney stones, menstrual cramps, migraines, muscle weakness, noise sensitivity, obesity, PMS, reflux, sleep disorders, and tremors.

Now I will review some of the key research done on the importance of magnesium for health and longevity.

MAGNESIUM AND ENERGY

In the May 2002 issue of the Journal of Nutrition, a study illustrated the ill effects of low magnesium levels on energy metabolism. This study showed inadequate magnesium was associated with a need for increased oxygen during exercise. Even during moderate activity, those with the lowest levels of magnesium in their muscles were likely to use more energy, and tire faster, than those with adequate levels.

Subjects were put on a diet providing adequate magnesium for 35 days, then switched to a diet providing less than half of the Recommended Daily Intake (RDI; formerly RDA) of magnesium, for 93 days. Finally, they were given adequate magnesium for the last phase of 49 days. A battery of tests was performed on the subjects at the end of each time period, including exercise tests, as well as biochemical and physiological tests.

Following the low magnesium phase, subjects had fewer red blood cells, and lower levels of magnesium stored in their muscles. They also used up more oxygen during exercise, and their heart rates jumped up about 10 beats per minute more. "When the volunteers were low in magnesium, they needed more energy and more oxygen to do low-level activities than when they were in adequate magnesium status," said Henry Lukaski, one of the study authors.

This study was not the first to indicate the body has to work harder if it is deficient in magnesium—and this applies to anyone with low magnesium, whether they are athletic or sedentary. For the average person, adequate magnesium levels are required just to make sure their heart and muscles have enough energy for daily living. For the athlete, good magnesium levels are required for going the distance in exercising, training, and sports performance.

MAGNESIUM AND THE ATHLETE

The body uses magnesium when dealing with stress, and the higher the stress, whether physical, emotional, or mental, the more magnesium the body will use up. Athletes are under immense amounts of all kinds of stress, and so have even higher requirements than the average person. In fact, serious athletes are often found to be deficient in magnesium, which can be easily corrected through supplementation.

Magnesium is required for post-exercise muscle recovery, after any athletic endeavor. Since severe magnesium deficiency is associated with structural damage to muscle cells, studies done on athletes show the higher their magnesium stores were, the better muscle integrity and function they had.

Another factor that will cause magnesium loss in the athlete is profuse sweating. Sweating from physical activity, or just undue heat, is going to contribute to magnesium loss, since magnesium—unlike most minerals—is highly water-soluble. It is perhaps the most important of the electrolytes we lose through excessive sweating (or fluid loss during illness), since it is the mostly commonly deficient one. As we sweat out magnesium, the percentage of calcium remaining in the blood will rise, and since calcium is a muscle contractor, muscle cramping is again likely to occur, if our body is lacking magnesium. One study found an 86% reduction in muscle cramps, when swimmers were given magnesium supplements during training and competition.

MAGNESIUM AND HEART DISEASE

About one of every three deaths in North America is due to cardiovascular disease and stroke, and magnesium deficiency is proven to cause angina, arrhythmia, and heart palpitations. If you are in a hospital with life threatening arrhythmia, doctors will use intravenous magnesium to save your life, but, unfortunately, they will never suggest you take it as a supplement to prevent heart disease in your future.

A study, published in the American Journal of Clinical Nutrition (March 2002), found an association between diets low in magnesium and irregular heartbeats. This study provided 22 postmenopausal women with a diet of conventional foods, containing either less than half of the RDI for magnesium, or more than the RDI for magnesium (320 mg daily). The volunteers ate both controlled diets (each diet for 81 days), but were not told which diet they were eating during any given phase of the study. After each diet phase, their magnesium levels were measured through blood tests, and electro-cardiograms were taken to measure the volunteers' heart rhythms.

When these women ate a diet containing just 40% of the RDI for magnesium, they all showed signs of magnesium deficiency in their blood serum, red blood cells, and urine. As well, they showed small increases in heartbeats that arise in abnormal areas within the heart. These are called ectopic heartbeats, and indicate increased myocardial danger. No such dangers were observed during the phase when they received adequate magnesium. Of course, if one is experiencing arrhythmia, the wise thing to do is start on a therapeutic dose of magnesium, not simply hope one can acquire sufficient magnesium from food.

A stronger indicator of potential heart disease than either high, or imbalanced (HDL to LDL ratio), cholesterol levels, is a benchmark of inflammation called C-reactive protein. Magnesium deficiency can cause general inflammation in the body, as well as higher C-reactive protein levels. (4)

Animal and human studies also indicate magnesium plays an important role in preventing ischemic heart disease (IHD), caused by blocked or narrowed arteries. Data from a population study (25-75 year old participants, followed for 20 years) were used to examine the association between serum magnesium concentration, and mortality from IHD, or all causes. Their conclusion was, "Serum magnesium concentrations were inversely associated with mortality from IHD and all-cause mortality". (5)

Regarding strokes, one study suggests low blood levels of magnesium can increase stroke risk by 25%. This study analyzed over 14,000 men and women, between the ages of 45 and 64, over the course of 15 years. The results indicated "higher serum magnesium levels were associated with lower prevalence of hypertension and diabetes mellitus". This study concluded it was this reduction in high blood pressure, and diabetes, which led to a reduced risk of stroke. (6)

MAGNESIUM AND INSULIN RESISTANCE

Both diabetes and metabolic syndrome are conditions of aberrant blood sugar metabolism, and are associated with a greater risk of cardiovascular disease, among other ailments. Other studies also strongly suggest magnesium may provide protection against diabetes, as well as metabolic syndrome.

Metabolic syndrome is the current name for insulin resistance, and is essentially a pre-diabetic condition. It describes a situation in which fat, the liver, or muscle tissues, can no longer properly respond to insulin's signal to bring glucose into cells. Since insulin resistance causes a wide range of ailments—from hypoglycemia and abdominal fat, to Alzheimer's disease—it is a condition we all need to pay attention to.

During conditions of insulin resistance, glucose and triglyceride levels rise in the blood, while high-density lipoprotein (HDL, the good cholesterol) declines—leading to hardening of the arteries—and blood pressure rises. In a study of more than 1,000 healthy adults, over a period of five years, researchers found that greater magnesium intake improved insulin sensitivity. (7) According to recent research, magnesium could correct several components of metabolic syndrome by increasing levels of HDL, decreasing triglycerides, and improving glucose homeostasis, insulin action, and insulin secretion. (8)

As mentioned above (in the section on heart disease), increased magnesium intake also protects against hypertension, another symptom of metabolic syndrome. While there are not much data to support the use of magnesium to treat high blood pressure, I have seen many cases where a low calcium regimen, in combination with therapeutic doses of magnesium, can bring blood pressure back to within healthy parameters, quickly and safely.

DIABETES

A diet abundant in magnesium-rich foods can substantially reduce risk of developing type 2 diabetes, according to a report from Harvard University. Researchers followed 85,000 women, and 42,000 men, for almost two decades. Even among subjects with an increased risk for diabetes—based on factors such as excess weight, little physical activity, and smoking—those with the highest levels of dietary magnesium intake, reduced their risk of developing type 2 diabetes by over 30%. (9)

Magnesium deficiency in diabetics can also cause complications such as eye disease (retinopathy), kidney disease (nephropathy), nerve disease (neuropathy), and foot ulcerations. Clearly, individuals who have diabetes should pay close attention to their magnesium status, in order to avoid these dangerous symptoms of the disease.

MAGNESIUM AND THE BRAIN

Researchers from Massachusetts Institute of Technology reported magnesium appears to be essential for maintaining memory function as we age. They discovered magnesium regulates key brain receptors required for learning and memory.

"Our study shows that maintaining proper magnesium in the cerebrospinal fluid is essential for maintaining the plasticity of synapses. Since it is estimated that the majority of American adults consume less than the estimated average requirement of magnesium, it is possible that such a deficit may have detrimental effects, resulting in potential declines in memory function." (10)

The ability of the brain to change is defined as "plasticity", and is critical to the ability to learn and remember. Aging and diseased brains lose synaptic plasticity. When this occurs in the hippocampus, where short-term memory is stored, we experience forgetfulness.

In the same study, they found increasing serum magnesium concentrations "led to the largest increases of plasticity ever reported in scientific literature". These findings indicate a deficiency in

K.W. PETERS

magnesium can impair learning and memory. While, on the other hand, providing the body with more magnesium than is required for its basic needs, may improve cognitive function. Scientists have even found magnesium helps speed recovery of cognitive function, following experimentally induced brain injury in lab animals. This suggests it would be a good idea to take a therapeutic dose of magnesium following a stroke, or for any other kind of brain damage.

Magnesium also plays a role in neurotransmitter release, which means it is necessary simply in order to maintain a healthy mood. A positive mood is a precursor to a balanced lifestyle, which in turn is part of maintaining a healthy brain. So, it is pretty clear maintaining high magnesium levels in the body is an important strategy for preventing memory decline, impaired learning, and senile dementia, which often accompanies aging.

MAGNESIUM BATHS

In 1618, a farmer from Epsom, England, found his cows would not drink from a certain well, because of the bitter taste of the water. He also noticed the water seemed to have a healing effect on the skin. As word spread, the dried substance from that well became known as Epsom salts, and eventually was determined to be magnesium sulfate.

These days, we take a bath with Epsom salts to relax the muscles and calm the body, but, done right, it can also increase our blood-levels of magnesium. For this to occur, one must add about two cups of Epsom salts to a hot bath, and stew in there for at least 20 minutes.

Magnesium is well absorbed through the skin, so Epsom salts, and "magnesium oil", are valid ways of increasing your body's store of magnesium. For some people, topical absorption is preferred over oral supplementation, especially if they are sensitive to the digestive disturbances that magnesium can cause—namely a laxative effect. Some will use magnesium as a safe laxative, but those with bowel conditions such as IBS, colitis, or Crohn's disease, may find they get the laxative effect before absorbing sufficient magnesium for the daily needs of their body. By taking magnesium in through the skin, they can avoid this unpleasant side effect.

MAGNESIUM OIL

Since the topical forms of magnesium have become more popular, there is now a variety of transdermal magnesium products on the market. Some are referred to as "Magnesium Oil", though they are not actually oils, being made from concentrated magnesium chloride, extracted from seawater. However, since the substance has the same viscous feel as oil, it has been given that name (or, sometimes, it is just referred to as liquid magnesium chloride). Another variation of topical magnesium is made from Epsom salts (Epsom Gel), and is in the form of magnesium sulfate rather than chloride. These two substances are both colorless and odorless, and work pretty much the same.

The topical application of magnesium is second only to intravenous delivery for quickly raising blood levels. Another advantage of topical magnesium is we can quickly target areas that are in need of magnesium. This is faster than waiting for a supplement to pass through the digestive system, enter the bloodstream, and find its way to the location where it is required.

Thus, we can rub the oil or gel directly on the legs if they are cramping, onto sore joints, onto the belly for menstrual cramps, or onto the chest if the heartbeat is irregular. To target the lymph system (part of our detoxification pathways), apply magnesium oil to the armpits, behind the knees, and on top of the feet. Really massaging it into the skin in these areas will encourage faster absorption.

The one downside to topical use of magnesium is the stinging, or tingling, feeling many people experience, along with a slight rash. This is harmless, and is a result of magnesium penetrating the skin. Usually, if you mix the "oil" with purified water in a 50/50 ratio, this sensation will be mostly avoided. The suggested use of this 50/50 mix is to spray the whole body (ideally after a bath or shower, when the pores are open and receptive) with about 12 sprays—which can be done daily, if one so desires. After being sprayed on, the magnesium liquid can be rubbed into the skin for faster absorption, or just left to air dry. Later, after 20 or 30 minutes, if one does not like the slightly tacky feeling, it can be rinsed off, since most of the magnesium will have been absorbed by then.

OTHER BENEFITS OF TOPICAL MAGNESIUM

Product information from suppliers of magnesium oil suggests it may be used as a deodorant for armpits and feet, and can be used to brush the teeth, where it may help with gingivitis, halitosis, and plaque prevention. Some anecdotal information also implies brushing with magnesium liquid can help prevent cavities, and can aid in regenerating tooth enamel.

Those with arthritis have often found magnesium oil to offer fast relief from pain, and, when used regularly, to improve the long-term health of the afflicted joints. Magnesium oil has also been helpful for those suffering from fibromyalgia, providing quick relief from their pain.

Topical magnesium may also help rejuvenate damaged or wrinkled skin, and there is anecdotal evidence that, with regular use, it can reduce the appearance of age spots. Other skin ailments can also benefit from topical application, including acne, boils, and pimples. These will be disinfected, and will dry out, when targeted with full strength magnesium oil a few times daily. According to product literature, massaging magnesium oil into the scalp every night can, theoretically, reduce balding areas, and restore graying hair to its original color.

MAGNESIUM SUPPLEMENTS

In the U.S., the current RDI for magnesium is 320 mg for women over 31, and 420 mg for men over that age. However, many natural health experts now recommend their patients try to get at least 500 mg daily, and 600 mg, or more, for therapeutic purposes.

While magnesium supplements are available in a variety of forms, some forms are better absorbed than others are. For example, the oxide form of magnesium is poorly absorbed, as are the chloride and sulfate forms, when taken orally (though the last two absorb well in a transdermal form). Currently, the best value for a well-absorbed form of magnesium, in oral supplemental form, whether liquid, powder, or pill, is the citrate form.

Magnesium citrate is the mostly widely used magnesium supplement because it is inexpensive, well absorbed, and, for most people, is less likely to have a laxative effect than the oxide form (unless you take too much). It is available in capsule or powder form, with the powder considered somewhat more bioavailable, especially when mixed into warm water, which creates an ionic solution. Ionic minerals, evidenced by being clear in liquid rather than milky, are the smallest particles available, and the easiest to absorb, especially for those with compromised digestion.

Other absorbable forms of magnesium include aspartate, glycinate (or bisglycinate), gluconate, malate, orotate, and taurate. These forms, like citrate, are simply bound to different salts, or amino acids, which serve to transport magnesium through the intestinal wall, and carry it throughout the body.

Though somewhat more expensive, the bisglycinate form is better absorbed than the citrate form, and appears to be retained longer. Magnesium bisglycinate is, currently, believed to be the best magnesium for general healing purposes, at a reasonable price point (again, with the powder being better absorbed than the capsules). Read the label well though, since many bisglycinate encapsulated products are mixed with the cheap oxide form of magnesium.

One form of magnesium particularly good for the heart is magnesium taurate, a combination of the amino acid taurine and magnesium. Since taurine is necessary for a strong heart muscle, binding it with magnesium creates a synergistic effect, which treats heart ailments more specifically than other forms of magnesium. (However, all forms of magnesium will still be of benefit to the heart.)

Magnesium malate is magnesium bound to malic acid, a weak organic acid found in vegetables and fruit. Malic acid is a key component of energy-creating chemical reactions in the body, making this the preferred form for treating chronic fatigue syndrome, and fibromyalgia.

A new form of magnesium, known as magnesium threonate, evidently has the ability to cross the blood-brain barrier, which makes it the best form for dealing with brain injury, dementia, mood disorders, and stroke damage. This form is quite expensive, but tends to be used at lower doses than other forms of magnesium.

Note that all figures used above (and below) refer to "elemental" numbers. Different forms of magnesium have different percentages of actual bioavailable (elemental) magnesium. Magnesium oxide is 60% elemental magnesium (but poorly absorbed), while other forms of magnesium will vary from 6.5% (malate) to 16% (citrate) elemental.

For example, 1000 mg of magnesium malate will only provide 65 mg of usable magnesium, whereas 1000 mg of magnesium citrate will provide about 160 mg of elemental magnesium. These figures will be on the label, when purchasing any reputable magnesium product.

MAGNESIUM AS A LAXATIVE

If your only need for magnesium is as a laxative, the poorly absorbed oxide form of magnesium will work just fine, providing an inexpensive alternative to habit-forming drugstore laxatives. Be aware, however, that high doses of poorly absorbed magnesium (consumed long-term), can put a strain on the kidneys, if they are already weak.

As well, remember even the well-absorbed forms of magnesium will have a laxative effect if you take too much. To prevent a laxative effect, the general rule of thumb (for those not overly sensitive to magnesium) is to take no more than 300 mg at once, and no more than 600 mg in a day.

While constipation can be caused by too much calcium (due to its constrictive nature), a deficiency in magnesium can also contribute to this problem. Of course, sometimes constipation is caused by more complicated issues, such as being a side effect of certain medications (like opiates). In these cases, magnesium can be used as a safe laxative, with the bonus of offering some nutritive value.

Usually, taking 400 to 500 mg of elemental magnesium oxide before bed, will give the desired response in the morning. If that does not work, try taking more, until a laxative effect is obtained.

The more expensive magnesium-based products marketed as laxatives, or bowel cleansers, usually contain magnesium hydroxide. Like the oxide form, it has a low solubility in water (leading to poor absorption), which causes it to draw water from the surrounding tissues by osmosis, thereby creating the laxative effect. When suspended in water, it is known as milk of magnesia, and is marketed as both a laxative and an antacid.

HOW TO TAKE MAGNESIUM

Magnesium stores are lowest in the early morning (often when leg or foot cramps occur), and late afternoon. Since many people find magnesium aids in getting a good night's sleep (due to its relaxing and anti-stress properties), the best times to take magnesium are before bed, and in the morning.

Generally, magnesium can be taken with, or without, food, but, if it is being used therapeutically, it is preferable to take it between meals for better absorption. The exception is magnesium oxide, which requires stomach acid to be broken down and assimilated. So, unless it is being used as a laxative, magnesium oxide should be taken with food.

However, the oxide form can act as an antacid, so for those with weak digestion, magnesium oxide, if taken with meals, may neutralize stomach acid, and further impair digestion. For those with poor digestion, the citrate and malate forms, being more acidic in nature, would be better to take with food.

If you get diarrhea, or loose stools, while taking magnesium, it usually means you are taking too much at one time. When taking a therapeutic dose (600 mg or more), be sure to space it out through the day. Most people are fine with 300 mg twice daily, but if that appears to be too much, divide the dose into smaller amounts, taken three or four times per day. If that does not improve things, you may need to cut back the total amount you are taking, or try switching to another form of magnesium.

Some people have a poor response with magnesium citrate or malate, because of the acidic nature of these forms, so an adverse reaction may simply mean you are taking a form that does not agree with your body. Of course, one can always resort to topical application, if supplements are intolerable.

FOODS HIGHEST IN MAGNESIUM

Assuming you have none of the risk factors leading to depleted magnesium levels (listed below), diet alone can prevent magnesium deficiency—and even correct a slight deficiency. This approach has the advantage of improving general health, since most of the foods high in magnesium are part of an overall healthy diet.

However, since the majority of food consumed in North America is over-processed, much of what passes for food these days is depleted of most of its vitamin and mineral content. As well, over-cooking also removes magnesium from food, and non-organically grown food is lacking in magnesium. Therefore, it can be hard to replenish entirely through diet alone, without focused attention on what we are eating. Thus, in many cases, magnesium supplements may be required to get stores back up, before relying solely on diet.

"Hard" water (which is high in minerals) can be a source of magnesium, but amounts of magnesium varies dramatically, depending on where the water is sourced from. Bottled waters from springs and glaciers will usually contain magnesium, and many purified waters add magnesium to their products. In either case, the label will give an indication of how much magnesium is present.

Certain fish can be a good source of magnesium, as any fish high in omega-3 fatty acids is also high in magnesium. The other foods with the highest magnesium content include, almonds, avocado, barley, beans, brown rice, buckwheat, dark leafy greens, dates, dulse, figs, garlic, kelp, legumes, millet, nuts, parsley, rye, soybeans, tofu, wheat germ, and whole grains. All these foods will be much higher in magnesium if they are grown organically and unrefined.

WHAT DEPLETES MAGNESIUM?

Anything that depletes magnesium levels is going to hurt us in the long run, so let's have a look at what things we should be wary of.

- Stress alone depletes magnesium, but stress can also result in decreased stomach acid. Decreased hydrochloric acid in the stomach results in decreased absorption of magnesium from foods. Low stomach acid can also be indicated by symptoms of reflux and heartburn (the same symptoms caused by high stomach acid), and by thick ridges on the thumbnail.

- Drinking "soft" water (water low in minerals or acidic in nature) consistently, will deplete magnesium. This includes distilled and reverse osmosis waters that are not re-mineralized.

- A diet high in acidic foods (excess animal protein, refined carbohydrates, sugars, processed foods, excess salt), will deplete the body of magnesium, along with many of the other minerals necessary for good health.

- Certain nutrients require magnesium for their proper assimilation. Nutrients that need magnesium include vitamins A, B2, B12, D, C, E, K, biotin, folic acid, and the minerals calcium, copper, iron, potassium, and zinc. So, if we are taking these nutrients as supplements—which are amounts higher than food provides—we should ensure that magnesium is among the mix.

- Synthetic fluoride in water and toothpaste binds to magnesium (making it unavailable to the body), and replaces magnesium in bone and cartilage.

- People with certain health problems like Crohn's disease, alcoholism, gluten-sensitivity or celiac disease, and hyperglycemia, may have higher magnesium requirements than the general population.

VITAMIN D AND MAGNESIUM

We know vitamin D works with vitamins A and K to build bones and teeth, and with vitamin A and iodine to maintain and repair mucous membranes. There is one other important cofactor which works with vitamin D, and that is magnesium.

Vitamin D uses magnesium to convert it from the inactive form to the active form, thereby "stealing" magnesium from the body. This is not a problem if you have plenty of magnesium stores in your body.

However, since magnesium deficiency is already widespread, what often happens is people start taking high levels of vitamin D only to find that it causes negative symptoms. Such symptoms may be due to worsening their pre-existing magnesium deficiency. In fact, if taking vitamin D supplements does not raise your blood levels of D, it may be because there is not sufficient magnesium in your body to facilitate its conversion into the active form.

Here is a list of symptoms experienced by some people taking high amounts of vitamin D: anxiety, constipation, headaches, heart palpitations, insomnia, muscle cramps, and increased pain levels in the bones or body. These are all also symptoms of magnesium deficiency. Thus, if you experience these symptoms while taking vitamin D, and you are not already supplementing with magnesium, it may be a good idea to try adding magnesium to your regimen before you give up on D.

PHARMACEUTICALS

Research has indicated that surgery done without increasing magnesium levels first, is more dangerous than surgery done when magnesium is administered before, during, and afterwards. So, when facing surgery, it would be wise to stay on top of your magnesium levels.

Almost all prescription drugs lead to a gradual depletion of vitamins, minerals and/or other essential nutrients from the body. Therefore, it is no surprise that many pharmaceutical drugs dangerously deplete magnesium levels.

Currently the U.S. FDA is informing the public that prescription Proton Pump Inhibitor drugs (which block stomach acid) may cause low serum magnesium levels, if taken for prolonged periods of time (usually longer than one year).

Specific drugs that cause magnesium depletion include, alcohol, antibiotics, anticonvulsants, anti-diabetics (oral), antihistamines, aspirin, beta-adrenergic agonists (for asthma), birth control pills, cocaine, corticosteroids, diuretics, insulin, nicotine, and cisplatin (which is used to treat cancer).

WARNINGS

Individuals with kidney failure lose the ability to remove excess magnesium from the blood. Such individuals should therefore carefully monitor magnesium supplementation, due to risk of magnesium toxicity—especially if they are using high amounts daily for laxative purposes.

Symptoms of excess magnesium can include appetite loss, diarrhea, muscle weakness, nausea, and extremely low blood pressure. Those with kidney problems should use the topical form of magnesium, after consulting with a health professional.

CONCLUSION

It is obvious that we have reams of scientific data supporting the use of magnesium to prevent—and in many cases even reverse—a wide range of modern ailments. That a doctor never discusses this essential nutrient with patients faced with any of the discussed ailments is a sad commentary on the current medical system. As well, it is an indication of how divorced the medical system is from the rest of the scientific community. After all, these are peer reviewed, double blind, truly scientific studies, which are, supposedly, exactly what the medical profession is based on.

Endnotes

1. Tong, GM, et al. 2005. "Magnesium deficiency in critical illness." J Intensive Care Med 20.
2. Rosanoff A, Weaver CM, Rude RK. Suboptimal magnesium status in the United States: are the health consequences underestimated? Nutr Rev. 2012 Mar.
3. Tucker KL, et al. "Potassium, magnesium, and fruit and vegetable intakes are associated with greater bone mineral density in elderly men and women." Am J Clin Nutr. 1999 Apr.
4. J Am Coll Nutr. 2005 Jun; 24(3):166-71. "Dietary magnesium and C-reactive protein levels." King DE, et al, Medical University of South Carolina.
5. Int J Epidemiol. 1999 Aug; 28(4):645-51."Serum magnesium and ischaemic heart disease: findings from a national sample of US adults." Centers for Disease Control and Prevention, Atlanta, GA.
6. Am J Epidemiol. 2009 Jun 15; 169(12): "Serum and dietary magnesium and risk of ischemic stroke: the Atherosclerosis Risk in Communities Study." Ohira T1, et al.
7. Ma B, Lawson AB, et al. "Dairy, magnesium, and calcium intake in relation to insulin sensitivity: approaches to modeling a dose-dependent association." Am J Epidemiol. 2006 Sep.

8. He K, et al. "Magnesium intake and the metabolic syndrome: epidemiologic evidence to date." J Cardiometab Syndr. 2006 Fall.
9. Lopez-Ridaura R, et al. "Magnesium intake and risk of type 2 diabetes in men and women." Diabetes Care. 2004 Jan.
10. Slutsky I, et al. "Enhancement of synaptic plasticity through chronically reduced Ca^{2+} flux during uncorrelated activity." Neuron. 2004 Dec.

CHAPTER FIVE

MELATONIN

I believe having adequate levels of the hormone melatonin in our bodies is critical to staying healthy in modern times. Melatonin deficiency is rampant in our world due to two primary factors: artificial light and electromagnetic pollution—both of which inhibit normal melatonin synthesis in the body. This has led to widespread insomnia, and worse. Melatonin also serves as a powerful antioxidant, one that specifically works to prevent cancer, and has a multitude of other important functions in the body, quite aside from just helping us to sleep well. Therefore, I feel it is essential to supplement with melatonin, in order to compensate for an environment that is drastically depleting it.

WHAT IS MELATONIN?

Melatonin is a hormone secreted by our pineal gland (a small, pine cone-shaped gland about the size of a pea), buried deep inside the brain. Melatonin production peaks at night, and its primary purpose is to regulate the sleep cycles by influencing circadian rhythm—our internal biological clock. The circadian rhythm regulates the sleep/wake cycle, as well as body temperature, endocrine function, and some disease processes.

Acquiring between 7 and 9 hours of proper sleep nightly is essential to allow the body to repair, and maintain those bodily functions that keep us healthy and vibrant. Unlike sleep drugs, which can disrupt REM (dreaming) sleep, melatonin can restore both dreaming, and normal sleep patterns.

Most of our melatonin is produced by the pineal gland daily, if we spend at least a couple of hours outside (in daylight). However, its production is inhibited by artificial light, when we are trying to sleep—hence our need to sleep in a room that is as dark as possible. Small amounts of melatonin are also provided by our diet, via certain fruits and vegetables. In fact, a few years ago, when melatonin was not legally available in Canada, some companies were selling cherry extracts as a sleep aid, due to their naturally high melatonin content.

Synthetic melatonin is commonly available as a supplement now (even in Canada). This form is effective, and considered very safe, unlike the original products, which were extracted from the pineal glands of cows (now considered a dubious source, due to mad cow disease). For those who want a natural source of melatonin (rather than synthetic), one product on the market is made from pig pineal glands (because, so far, there is no mad pig disease). And recently, Bulletproof.com came out with a melatonin product extracted from plant sources (though it costs about 7 times more than synthetic melatonin).

EMFs AND MELATONIN

As will be covered in detail in part 3 of this book, one of the main dangers of the 21st century is our constant exposure to electromagnetic pollution. This comes in the form of electromagnetic radiation (cell phones and towers), radio frequencies (smart meters, wireless signals, cordless phones, baby monitors), and electromagnetic frequencies produced by electronic equipment and household wiring. For our purposes here, the important thing to note is that both animal and human studies have indicated that electromagnetic pollution reduces melatonin levels. (1)

A reduction in melatonin levels was found in people affected by the Schwarzenburg cell phone tower in Switzerland, but when the transmitter was shut down, their levels of melatonin gradually returned to normal. (2)

Another example occurred when German citizens in Lindauerstrabe took it upon themselves to observe and test the effects of a cell phone tower placed in their community. They took blood samples in November 2006, a month before the transmitter began operation. The second set of blood samples were taken 5 months after the transmitter commenced operating.

Results showed melatonin levels decreased in the presence of cell phone tower signal exposure, to nearly half of the normal level, for over half of the group. As well, 84% of participants reacted with an average decrease of about 46% in their serotonin levels, following exposure to the newly erected telecommunications tower. (3)

MELATONIN AND SEROTONIN

Melatonin produces some serotonin (our main calming neurotransmitter), and serotonin produces some melatonin, therefore when melatonin declines, serotonin in turn also declines. Low serotonin leads to increased anxiety, which raises levels of the stress hormone cortisol, which in turn can lead to an increased risk of diabetes, heart disease, and hypertension.

Serotonin is necessary for a sense of well-being, thus low serotonin levels can cause agitation, anxiety, depression, lethargy, and psychiatric disturbances. (Though, as we will see in the chapter on negative ions, excessively high levels of serotonin can create other problems.)

Considering the massive amount of electromagnetic pollution we are exposed to daily, we can look forward to increases in mental health problems throughout the population. These problems range from nameless anxiety and panic attacks, to road rage, domestic violence, and child abuse. We are already seeing an increase in these aberrant behaviors, and will continue to see an increase in all conditions where we need the inhibitory neurotransmitter serotonin to prevent us from acting out violent, or socially inappropriate, behaviors.

MELATONIN AS AN ANTIOXIDANT

While melatonin itself functions as a powerful antioxidant, it also helps to increase the levels and activity of two other antioxidants produced by the body: SOD (superoxide dismutase) and glutathione peroxidase.

Over and above its function of protecting against free radical damage in the body, SOD also serves as an anti-inflammatory, and works to repair damaged cells. This link between SOD and cell repair is illustrated by clinical studies, which have found an association between low levels of SOD and Lou Gehrig's disease (ALS), a condition that damages nerve cells in the brain and spinal cord.

In fact, research has found higher levels of ALS in those working in jobs that expose them to excessively high, consistent electromagnetic fields: "Nine out of the ten epidemiological studies that have been conducted on the risk of ALS in relation to occupational exposure to EMF show moderate to strong relative risk estimates that supported a link between them." (4) So, one could hypothesize that electromagnetic fields deplete melatonin from those workers exposed to them, which in turn leads to low SOD levels, reducing the ability of their bodies to repair damaged cells.

As mentioned above, melatonin also increases glutathione production in the body. This internally generated antioxidant is found in every cell of the body. And, as well as fighting free radicals, and repairing damage done by them, glutathione also serves to detoxify the cells. It is well established glutathione levels are seriously depleted in people with life-threatening diseases, including AIDS and cancer. Melatonin benefits glutathione levels by helping to recycle it, after it has given up its electron to neutralize a free radical.

MELATONIN AND CANCER

Throughout the world, where electricity is commonly used, light exposure during the night is becoming progressively commonplace. Artificial light has allowed humans to work throughout the 24-hour day, but, as photographs taken from outer space have indicated, it is also apparent that true darkness is disappearing from the "civilized" parts of the planet.

Until recently, we believed light pollution and night work were not an issue, in terms of human health, but this is no longer the case. Light at night is proven to disrupt circadian rhythms, and to suppress melatonin production.

Human population studies, and experimental animal studies, have shown one of the dangers of nighttime melatonin inhibition is cancer initiation and growth. Certain cancers are on the increase among individuals who routinely work nightshifts, or whose circadian rhythms are disrupted regularly for other reasons (such as repeated jet lag). The cancers related to melatonin inhibition include breast, colorectal, endometrial, and prostate. (5)

In 2005, a link between artificial light and breast cancer was reported in the December issue of the scientific journal Cancer Research. A study done with mice, revealed that exposing them to artificial light at night both suppressed melatonin levels, and stimulated the growth of breast tumors—whereas, if the periods of darkness were extended the growth of these tumors was slowed. This study might explain why female night shift workers have higher rates of breast cancer, and why industrialized countries are experiencing an epidemic rise in breast cancer rates.

"The risk of developing breast cancer is about five times higher in industrialized nations than it is in underdeveloped countries," said Les Reinlib, Ph.D., an administrator of the study. "These results suggest that the increasing nighttime use of electric lighting, both at home and in the workplace, may be a significant factor."

Further support for this thesis came from a nationwide

population-based, case-controlled study, investigating breast cancer risk among Danish women, between the ages of 30 and 54, who worked predominantly at night. In this study, those night shift workers had a breast cancer rate 1.5 times the rate of the day shift workers. (6)

Since breast cancer is a hormone-related form of cancer, it comes as no surprise to discover a link between artificial light and prostate cancer. A study from the University of Haifa, working with the University of Connecticut, examined the influence of artificial light at night on the incidence of lung, intestinal, and prostate cancers, in men from 164 different countries.

The researchers divided the countries into three groups: those with little exposure to lighting at night, those with medium exposure, and those with high exposure. In those countries with low exposure to nighttime light, the prostate cancer rate was about 67 incidents per 100,000 people. In those countries with medium exposure, the rate of prostate cancer went up 30% to about 87 occurrences per 100,000 inhabitants. Finally, in the countries with the highest level of exposure to artificial light at night, prostate cancer rates jumped up 80% to 157 patients per 100,000 people. The researchers suggested that increased incidence of prostate cancer, due to exposure to light at night, could be due to suppression of melatonin production.

All this data supports work done in Italy years ago, linking low melatonin levels to increased cancer rates. Some studies have even found melatonin supplementation to be an effective co-agent for treating cancers. Recently, Italian physicians have used melatonin along with conventional chemotherapy, and results showed better tumor regression, fewer side effects, and longer life, compared to those patients not receiving melatonin.

If this link between light exposure and cancer risk were accepted by industry, it could have a positive effect on the production and use of artificial lighting. For example, lighting that mimics sunlight (known as full-spectrum lighting) has been available for quite some time now, and could be used far more widely. Yet, more than just

K.W. PETERS

using light that supports melatonin production, we also need a new generation of lighting that prevents it from being blocked.

BLUE LIGHT

David Blask, M.D., a neuro-endocrinologist with the Bassett Research Institute, suggested that, "day workers who spend their time indoors would benefit from lighting that better mimics sunlight. Companies that employ shift workers could introduce lighting that allows the workers to see without disrupting their circadian and melatonin rhythms".

When the Sleep Research Centre at the University of Surrey (UK) did a study confirming light exposure at night suppressed melatonin levels, they also found something else. They looked at the composition of the spectral waves in the light, and found the actual color range of the light being used, in part, determined how deeply one slept and how long it took to attain deep sleep. (Deep sleep, or delta waves, is the level at which the body fully rests and restores.)

The researchers examined the blue-sensitive photoreceptors in the retina, which controls the pineal gland. When the blue-sensitive photoreceptors were exposed to blue light at night, the pineal gland was observed to suppress melatonin production. They concluded that, if we used lights with little or no blue content, we could eliminate the damaging effects of nighttime lighting. (7)

Many years before this study, scientists at John Carroll University developed special light bulbs that do not produce the blue wavelength (which causes melatonin suppression). As well, they developed eyeglasses that blocked blue light. Three of the scientists involved in this study left the university in 2005, and started a company to market these special light bulbs and glasses. They also developed and market blue-blocking filters for computer screens, TVs, and other electronic devices.

They called their company Photonic Developments, and their products, along with research articles, are available from their website at www.lowbluelights.com. This company is so confident their products will improve sleep patterns they offer a money-back guarantee.

One other option for reducing blue light is a software application for computers, laptops, smart phones, and tablets, known as f.lux. (Though currently not allowed on Apple products, they have their own version of this app called Night Shift.)

Computer (and other) monitors are designed to mimic daytime sunlight, which can be a problem when used late into the evening.

The f.lux program was designed specifically to reduce eyestrain during nighttime use, and reduce blue light disruption of sleep patterns. It does this by adjusting a display's color temperature, according to location and time of day.

Although the program itself has not been scientifically tested to determine its efficacy, f.lux has been widely, and positively, reviewed by technology journalists, bloggers, and users. (www.justgetflux.com)

Red light suppresses melatonin the least, so if we need a light for getting up at night to use the bathroom, a red nightlight is the best option. Remember, when you turn on a regular light at night, as far as your body is concerned the sun has just come up, and it accordingly reduces the amount of melatonin in your bloodstream. Which is why it can be hard to fall back to sleep afterwards. This rising at night to urinate is common to men, due to prostate swelling. However, when women have to get up frequently at night to urinate, studies have indicated it may be a result of melatonin deficiency.

EXCEPTION TO THE RULE

For most of us, the rule of light dissipating melatonin holds true, when it is used as a sleep agent. However, as we are seeing, melatonin has other functions as well, and there is a specific group of people that benefits from taking melatonin during the day—those suffering from seasonal affective disorder (SAD), a form of depression that occurs in the winter.

A study done at Oregon Health and Science University determined there were two types of patients suffering from SAD. One group, referred to as "phase-delayed types", or "night owls," responded best to taking low-dose melatonin in the afternoon or evening. The other group, known as "phase-advanced types", or "morning larks," responded best to taking low-dose melatonin in the morning.

For both groups, daytime use of melatonin alleviated SAD symptoms, and melatonin did not cause drowsiness, as the doses used were lower than amounts taken for sleeping purposes. (Unfortunately, the study synopsis I had access to did not define the doses.) (8)

Of course, those who work the night shift will also be taking their melatonin during the day. However, in this case, melatonin should be taken just before going to sleep (in a dark room), thereby tricking the body into thinking it is night.

NEUROLOGICAL DISORDERS

Declining levels of melatonin production, as we age, is one of the main contributing factors in the development of neuro-degenerative disorders. Studies have shown melatonin can prevent oxidative damage in both cultured neuronal cells, and in brains of animals treated with neuro-toxic agents.

These studies suggest melatonin may have a potential therapeutic effect in treating Alzheimer's, brain trauma, ALS, Huntington's disease, and stroke. As well, low levels of melatonin is somewhat linked to Parkinson's disease—though the science is not as strong as for the ailments previously listed.

It should be noted these types of studies use amounts of melatonin far above amounts recommended for maintaining healthy sleep patterns. The human equivalence of the amounts used in animal studies, and the actual amounts used in some human studies, range from

50 to 100 mg of melatonin. (9) However, these high levels should be used only under the guidance of a health professional.

MELATONIN AND LIVER HEALTH

The ability of melatonin to support liver health is illustrated by a rat study designed to compare melatonin to NAC (N-Acetyl Cysteine), a sulfur-bearing amino acid used for detoxification. In this study, researchers used methanol to injure the rats' livers, then studied the structural effects of these two liver-protective substances. Their conclusion was, "Melatonin is much more efficient than NAC, as well as significantly greater hepatoprotective effect against the liver injury secondary to the methanol intoxication". (10)

MELATONIN AND HEART DISEASE

Melatonin exerts control over fat-related metabolic functions in the body, so it is no surprise that studies (published in the Journal of Pineal Research) showed melatonin to have a positive effect on blood lipid profiles. In these studies, melatonin lowered triglycerides and LDL ("bad") cholesterol levels, while raising HDL ("good") cholesterol levels—all of which help to reduce risk of cardiovascular disease.

As mentioned at the beginning of this chapter, the primary purpose of melatonin is to regulate circadian rhythms. Not only do the circadian rhythms influence heart rate, they also affect blood pressure, and so can be involved in preventing strokes. Thus, via the mechanism of regulating circadian rhythms, melatonin contributes to protecting us from heart disease, hypertension, and stroke. Melatonin also protects us from these diseases though other mechanisms as well.

According to other studies from the Journal of Pineal Research, melatonin has antioxidant, anti-inflammatory, and gene-regulating functions that directly affect cardiovascular health. Many cardiac conditions are a result of free radical damage, and processes involving inflammation. Therefore, the beneficial effects of melatonin against these conditions were determined to be, in part, a result of its anti-oxidant properties. As well, other protective benefits of melatonin appear to be due to its function as an epigenetic regulator. Which is to say it has the ability to turn certain genes off or on, allowing them to express or not. (11)

MELATONIN AND BODY FAT

The ability of melatonin to regulate lipid (cholesterol/triglycerides) levels in the body can also work to regulate, and prevent, unhealthy weight gain. This was made evident in a Spanish study designed "to investigate the effects of melatonin on obesity and obesity-associated systolic hypertension and dyslipidemia in young male Zucker diabetic fatty rats".

The Spanish study was essentially an experimental model of metabolic syndrome, also known as insulin resistance. (Insulin resistance is a cause of diabetes, as well as unnatural weight gain.) In this study, the group receiving a melatonin supplement attained a significant reduction in body weight, without reducing calorie intake, compared to the placebo group. The authors of the study concluded that, "administration of melatonin and intake of food containing melatonin might be a useful tool to fight obesity and the risks associated with it". (12)

It is worth noting, the protective effects of melatonin shown in this study were more dramatic in younger subjects, before they developed insulin resistance, or vascular problems. This implies that melatonin supplementation should be started at an early age, in order to gain maximum health benefits.

MELATONIN AND LONGEVITY

Once we have moved past our prime in reproductive capability, sex hormones begin to decline. At this point, the pineal gland begins to atrophy, and the aging process kicks into full gear. Animal studies done at the Foundation for the Aged, in Italy, have indicated supplementing with melatonin can reverse this process of aging, to a great degree.

The work of Dr. Walter Pierpaoli, from the Foundation for the Aged, was summarized in his book "The Melatonin Miracle" (1995; Simon & Schuster Inc; NY, New York). Much of the material in this chapter, and the material to follow, on the subject of longevity, is based on this book—well worth a read for those who want the full story on melatonin.

Melatonin's value for promoting longevity is well illustrated by studies comparing aging in two groups of mice.

The original experiments involved transplanting pineal glands from young mice into old ones, and vice versa. Pineal glands from younger animals rejuvenated the older ones, and young mice given pineal glands from old mice rapidly aged, and died earlier than expected. Since the pineal gland is responsible for production of melatonin, the scientists later decided to see what would happen if they simply used the hormone, instead of transplanting glands.

In the new experiments, both groups of mice were aged. One group received melatonin in their nightly drinking water, and the other group received no melatonin. After 6 months, the untreated group aged as expected, losing hair in patches, shriveling, losing muscular coordination, suffering immune and thyroid degeneration, and eventually dying of cancer. (These were a cancer-prone breed, used in cancer research.)

On the other hand, the group of mice treated nightly with melatonin seemed to delay their aging process; they regained sexual vitality, their fur returned to a youthful level, and they lived about 30% longer than the control group.

The pineal gland also controls the immune system, so when it begins to run down, the immune system also begins to break down, leading to many of the symptoms of aging. Melatonin levels start their natural decline in humans at around the age of 45, but now this timetable is being accelerated, due to the effects of artificial light, and electromagnetic pollution.

WHO SHOULD NOT TAKE MELATONIN?

Clearly, melatonin deficiency is a 21st century issue, and something all adults should consider supplementing with, unless they live a country life with minimal electrical exposure. I say adults, because the one group that should not take melatonin is adolescents.

As mentioned in the beginning of this chapter, one of the main functions of melatonin is to regulate and run the endocrine system. The endocrine system is comprised of all the glands that produce hormones from infancy, and throughout our life. During the development of the sex organs, the body withholds melatonin, allowing other specific hormones to do their work moving the body into puberty. Doctors seem to be unaware of this, and often suggest that melatonin is suitable for children, and while small amounts may be safe for a while, by the time a child is approaching adolescence, it can be dangerous, and may impede sexual development.

A better approach for adolescents, and children, is to give them agents that increase levels of the neurotransmitter serotonin. Serotonin precursors, such as L-theanine, 5HTP (5-hydroxy tryptophan), and L-tryptophan, help to calm the nervous system, allowing one to easily fall asleep. Serotonin also serves as a precursor to melatonin, but will create no more than the optimal amount for their age.

One should also ensure young people get at least an hour (ideally more) of natural daylight outside, in order to allow the body to regulate its own melatonin production. Another solution for children, and adolescents, are the blue ray blocking glasses (mentioned previously under Blue Light). These glasses have been used on children, with good success, and no adverse effects.

For some reason (yet undefined), melatonin may cause excessive dreaming and/or nightmares, in certain people. It is important to note that we do not rest and restore when we are dreaming. Only deep "delta" wave sleep (which is dreamless) allows the body to repair and rejuvenate for the following day. Therefore, excessive dreaming can have a negative effect.

Those adults who have an adverse reaction to melatonin supplements can take the same approach that we use with children. They can increase their serotonin levels in order to elevate melatonin levels naturally. Both groups can also include foods that contain natural melatonin (which I will cover shortly).

Another approach to acquiring melatonin (without supplementation) is to eat foods high in the amino acid tryptophan, which is a precursor to serotonin. Foods high in tryptophan include almonds, chicken, dairy, pumpkin seeds, soy, spirulina, and turkey.

HOW MUCH MELATONIN DO YOU NEED?

One thing to be aware of when supplementing with melatonin is the amount that you require for your age. Most supplemental melatonin comes in 3 mg pills, yet, technically, only someone 70 years, or older, generally requires that much.

Taking too much melatonin can have the effect of keeping you awake, causing excessive dreaming, or leaving you feeling groggy in the morning. I generally suggest starting with 1 mg to 1.5 mg, sublingual (under the tongue), taken 5 minutes before shutting off the light. If that amount seems to have no effect, take 3 mg the next night, and, if again there is no response, try higher doses, until you find an effective dosage.

Melatonin is usually taken in a sublingual form, because it is easily destroyed by stomach acid, when simply swallowed in a pill. Another effective approach is to use enteric-coated melatonin, which does not release until it reaches the intestinal tract. This form is essentially a timed-release product, and is superior for those who have little trouble falling asleep, but who often wake up in the middle of the night.

Generally, I suggest people do not take amounts of melatonin much higher than their biological requirements. However, clinical studies done with cancer patients, and other disease models, will often use levels of 50 to 100 mg, so there are no worries about overdosing on it. Nonetheless, when we consistently take in high amounts of a synthesized nutrient, especially a hormone, we eventually reduce the body's ability to produce its own. This is one reason I always suggest people cycle their supplements (or only take them 5 days a week), and the same holds true for melatonin.

AGE REQUIREMENTS FOR MELATONIN

According to the premiere scientific researcher on melatonin (Dr. Walter Pierpaoli), the following is the average melatonin requirements for different age groups. Ages 40 to 44—0.5 to 1 mg; ages 45 to 54—1 to 2 mg; ages 55 to 64—2 to 2.5 mg; ages 65 to 74—2.5 to 5 mg; ages 75 and over—3.5 to 5 mg.

It should be noted that, according to Harvard Medical School, taking aspirin on a regular basis reduces melatonin levels in the body.

ENDOGENOUS VS EXOGENOUS

There is one argument against continually using a melatonin supplement, articulated for me by Paul Pitchford, in his book "Healing with Whole Foods". His position (which I agree with) is that the major danger of taking hormone supplements is that we can become dependent on them. Which is why I suggested earlier that one not take them 7 days a week, instead trying to skip a couple of days each week, or cycling off and on, over time.

When a hormone is introduced into the body consistently, or in unnaturally high amounts, coming from outside the body (exogenous), it causes the body to reduce, or even cease, production of that hormone from within the body (endogenous).

This tendency of the body to reduce natural production of hormones has been observed in those taking hormone-replacement therapy—especially when the dosage has not been tuned precisely to the body's needs, through constant hormone testing.

The obvious example is steroid users, who take amounts of testosterone well in excess of natural human levels. When they stop taking it, their body can no longer produce the hormone internally, as the function has been usurped by taking too much externally provided testosterone. This is a further argument for only taking levels of hormones close to what our body would naturally provide, and not much more than that.

If we wish to err on the side of caution, we can use all the previously discussed methods for normalizing melatonin levels naturally: avoiding electromagnetic pollution, eating foods rich in tryptophan and melatonin, getting sufficient daylight on the face, and using blue blocking lenses or screens.

That being said, I, like most people, live in a highly unnatural environment—in a city, surrounded by cell phone towers, with every home using a smart meter, and every neighbor's wireless signals passing through my house. If the price I have to pay for city living is taking a small amount of melatonin under my tongue before bed—and the only side effect is potentially a longer life and maybe less disease—it is a price I am willing to pay.

NATURAL SOURCES OF MELATONIN

If we wish to follow Paul Pitchford's lead, and acquire our melatonin naturally from food sources, there are enough studies to indicate this is possible.

One study, done at Khon Kaen University in Thailand, showed certain tropical fruits were very effective at raising blood levels of melatonin. Testing done on 30 people, utilized six different tropical fruits, feeding subjects a large amount of one particular fruit for a week, followed by a week avoiding that fruit. During the study, the subjects' urine was analyzed for a metabolite of melatonin, which indicates higher blood levels of circulating melatonin.

Each fruit was tested in turn with the most dramatic rise in melatonin resulting from the consumption of bananas, oranges, and pineapples. Pineapples increased the melatonin metabolite levels by 266%, bananas by 180%, and oranges by 47%. (13) This may be one reason why bananas and oranges are two of the most popular fruits in the West.

As mentioned in the opening of this chapter, cherry juice can also be used as a natural way to raise melatonin levels. This is perhaps a better choice for those of us in the West, since it is not a tropical fruit (which tend to be high in sugar and more suited to the diet of those living in hot climates). The highest amount of melatonin is found in the tart cherry (Prunus cerasus, also known as Montmorency cherries). One study found that drinking tart cherry juice for a week increased the amount of sleep time in subjects by about 30 minutes, and provided a more restful sleep.

Other foods known to increase melatonin levels in the body include almonds, barley, cardamom, coriander, fennel, ginger, goji berries, mangosteen, mustard seeds, oats, rice, sunflower seeds, sweet corn, and tomatoes.

A WORD ABOUT FLUORIDE

I belong to the camp that believes fluoride is a toxic compound, which has no place in dentistry, or as an additive to drinking water. Fluoride is associated with cancer, diminished IQ, and thyroid and immune malfunction, among other ailments.

While there is naturally occurring fluoride, found in very small amount in some waters, and foods, this can also be said of cyanide and arsenic, yet no one suggests adding those to your drinking water.

I raise the subject of fluoride here because it also accumulates in the pineal gland, which produces our melatonin.

One scientist (Dr. Jennifer Luke), reflecting on the idea that the pineal gland is a calcifying tissue, hypothesized it might also store high levels of fluoride. To test this theory, she had the pineal gland of 11 cadavers analyzed, and found high levels of fluoride in the calcium hydroxyapatite crystals produced by the gland. The levels were (in some cases) higher than fluoride levels found in bones of patients suffering from skeletal fluorosis (a disease caused by excessive fluoride accumulation in bones). She further hypothesized that fluoride was inhibiting one of the enzymes needed by the body to convert the amino acid tryptophan into melatonin, resulting in an impaired production of this essential hormone.

As mentioned above, melatonin is responsible for triggering the onset of puberty—particularly the inhibition of melatonin at the right phase of sexual development. Knowing this, Dr. Luke conducted a gerbil study in which she discovered gerbils treated with high amounts of fluoride reached puberty earlier than those treated with low levels. This result confirmed her theory that fluoride was indeed inhibiting melatonin production to a significant degree. (14)

What we can take away from this is the knowledge that, if we wish to keep a healthy pineal gland, we need to avoid ingesting fluoride in fluoridated toothpaste, water, and dental treatments. And, especially, we should not expose children to this toxin.

In order to remove fluoride from our pineal gland, we need to take in a good amount of iodine. Fluoride is a halogen, and iodine is the most effective way to remove halogens from the body.

Endnotes

1. Radiat Prot Dosimetry. 2013 May; 154(4):405-16; "Pineal melatonin level disruption in humans due to electromagnetic fields and ICNIRP limits."

2. "Effect of short-wave (6-22 MHz) magnetic fields on sleep quality and melatonin cycle in humans: the Schwarzenburg shutdown study." Altpeter ES, et al; Bioelectromagnetics. 2006 Feb; 27(2):142-50

3. Germany: Study on residents near Mast shows alarming evidence of harm to health and wellbeing." www.mastsanity.org

4. Am J Ind Med. 2003 Feb; 43(2):212-20. "Association between occupational exposure to power frequency electromagnetic fields and amyotrophic lateral sclerosis: a review." Li CY, Sung FC.

5. Crit Rev Oncog. 2007 Dec; 13; "Light at night, chronodisruption, melatonin suppression, and cancer risk: a review." Reiter RJ, et al.

6. Epidemiology. 2001 Jan; 12 "Increased breast cancer risk among women who work predominantly at night." Hansen J., Danish Cancer Society

7. "The spectral composition of evening light and individual differences in the suppression of melatonin and delay of sleep in humans." – Santhi N, Thorne HC, et al; J Pineal Res. 2011 Sep 20

8. Oregon Health and Science University. "Melatonin Improves Mood In Winter Depression." ScienceDaily. ScienceDaily, 2 May 2006

9. Neurotox Res. 2012 Jun 28; "Melatonin Antioxidative Defense: Therapeutical Implications for Aging and Neurodegenerative Processes." Pandi-Perumal SR, et al.

10. Eur Rev Med Pharmacol Sci. 2012 Apr; 16; "Effect of melatonin and n-acetylcysteine on hepatic injury in rat induced by methanol intoxication: a comparative study." Koksal M, et al.

11. Melatonin and circadian biology in human cardiovascular disease; Journal of Pineal Research Volume 49, Issue 1, pp14–22, August 2010

12. Beneficial effects of melatonin on obesity and lipid profile in young Zucker diabetic fatty rats. Journal of Pineal Research, Volume 50, Issue 2, pp 207–212, March 2011

13. Johns NP, et al. "Dietary intake of melatonin from tropical fruit altered urinary excretion of 6-sulfatoxymelatonin in healthy volunteers." J Agric Food Chem. 2013 Jan 30; 61(4):913-9

14. The Effect of Fluoride on the Physiology of the Pineal Gland." Luke J. Ph.D Dissertation, School of Biological Sciences, University of Surrey, UK. 1997

SLEEP DISORDERS

Since both electromagnetic pollution, and artificial light at night, reduce our natural production of melatonin, it is little wonder insomnia is a growing problem. In this chapter, I will examine the natural approach to insomnia, covering both supplements and lifestyle adjustments.

SYMPTOMS OF SLEEP DEPRIVATION

If you have ever suffered from a sleep disorder, you are well aware of why prevention of sleep has been used as a highly effective torture technique. In modern times, it has been well documented chronic lack of sleep has a horrendous effect on health. Following are the main symptoms of sleep deprivation:

- Increased risk of diabetes, heart disease, hypertension, and stroke.

- Increased rates of accidents (both traffic and workplace).

- Impaired alertness, attention, concentration, learning, reasoning, and problem solving.

- Lowered libido in both genders.

- Increased risk of depression—those with insomnia are 5 times more likely to develop depression as those without it.

- Premature aging—lack of sleep causes an increase in the stress hormone cortisol, and excess cortisol can break down skin collagen (the protein that keeps skin smooth and unwrinkled). A lack of sleep also reduces production of human growth hormone (HGH), necessary for repairing the body as we age, maintaining muscle mass, and keeping bones strong.

- Weight gain—those who sleep fewer than six hours per day were shown in one study to be 30% more likely to become obese than those who slept seven to nine hours.

SLEEPING PILLS

If you are reading this book, the odds are you are the type of person to avoid taking prescription medications whenever possible. Like most medications, sleeping pills can have a variety of side effects. The most common side effect of the last generation of sleeping pills (benzodiazepines and barbiturates) is dependency—with the potential for addiction.

Some newer forms of sleeping pills (Lunesta, Sonata, and Ambien, for example), are "less likely to be habit forming". But, even these come with a list of potential side effects that should make us think twice before using them.

Here is a partial list of side effects from the newer sleeping pills: burning or tingling in the extremities, constipation, diarrhea, dizziness, daytime drowsiness, dry mouth or throat, headache, problems with attention or memory, tremors, and/or stomach pain.

When we treat insomnia naturally, only positive side effects occur. For example, the antioxidant and anti-carcinogenic properties of melatonin, and the immune-enhancing side effects of L-theanine.

Now, let's have a look at steps we can take to ensure we get a good night's sleep, on a regular basis.

ELECTROMAGNETIC POLLUTION

Try to minimize your evening exposure to electromagnetic pollution, in order to facilitate sleeping, and allow natural melatonin production to occur. Since we are exposed to high levels of these fields during our waking hours, it is important to give the body a break during the night.

During sleep, our body detoxifies and regenerates, so we want our bedrooms to have very low levels of electromagnetic pollution. Furthermore, in order to properly detoxify during sleep we must have an alkaline pH, and electromagnetic pollution creates acidity in the body.

EATING LATE

We should not eat for at least two or three hours before bed for a number of reasons. If the body has to pump blood to the digestive system in order to facilitate digestion, then the heart is working when it should be resting. This can leave us feeling tired in the morning, instead of refreshed.

If large amounts of simple carbohydrates are consumed within a few hours of bedtime, growth hormone production will decline (due to the ensuing spike in insulin), and the body will not be able to repair and restore efficiently. People usually crave carbohydrates in the evening because they produce serotonin in the body, promoting relaxation and drowsiness. However, it is preferable to use serotonin-precursor supplements (discussed further on), in order to avoid the side effects of eating carbohydrates before bed.

Finally, from the perspective of weight management, eating too many calories before bed is undesirable. Since sleeping is not an activity of a thermal nature, those calories cannot be burned up, and are likely to be stored as fat.

EXERCISE

Studies have shown there is a relationship between melatonin and the stress hormone, cortisol. In physical stress studies done on rats and humans, it was discovered vigorous exercise in the evening significantly increases cortisol levels. Cortisol will in turn dramatically reduce the normal nighttime surge of melatonin.

Normally, cortisol releases in a rhythmic pattern throughout the day—depending on circumstances. It is high in the morning, which gets us out of bed, and energized enough to begin the day. It is at its lowest level around 2 a.m., which is when melatonin is at its highest, and this inverse relationship allows the body to regenerate.

This regeneration process is impeded if nighttime cortisol levels are too high, because high cortisol breaks down tissue (catabolism). As well, high cortisol reduces the amounts of growth hormone, and thyroid-stimulating hormone, that we produce at night. Both of these hormones are necessary for the body to repair itself, allowing it to build new cells and tissues.

This ability for the body to heal and regenerate at night, is one of the most important reasons good sleep is essential to well being. And, it is known that people with high cortisol levels at night generally also have sleep disorders. Therefore, one should avoid doing vigorous exercise for a few hours before going to bed.

WHAT DIRECTION TO FACE WHEN SLEEPING

According to a variety of healing traditions, the direction of our head, while sleeping, can have a dramatic effect on how well we sleep, and how rested we feel the next day.

It is believed in the Western natural healing traditions that we sleep better if our head faces north. However, when I researched further, I found some conflicting ideas.

I am not sure where the idea of orienting north originated, but I would assume that it came from people observing animal behavior. Recently science supported this thesis, when researchers used

Google Earth satellite images to reveal herds of sleeping cattle almost exclusively face in the north-south direction of the Earth's magnetic lines.

Direct observations of almost 3,000 red and roe deer also showed those animals align their body axis in roughly a north-south direction—orienting their heads northward, during grazing and resting periods.

Both the cattle and the deer faced more in the magnetic north-south direction, rather than the geographic north-south direction. This is relevant since the Earth's magnetic poles do not line up perfectly with the North and South Poles as seen on maps ("true north"). Since there is roughly a twenty degree difference between true north and magnetic north, when choosing where to position your head, it is best to use a compass.

Facing north seemed reasonable, since we are (after all) mammals, but then I discovered the Ayurvedic (East Indian) tradition believes just the opposite. Their healing system advises we avoid sleeping with our head to the north or west, and that the best direction to face is east or south. And, they firmly believe it is downright unhealthy to sleep facing the wrong direction, because it can lead to mental and physical problems.

For those who follow the north-facing system, south is the worst direction to face because the mind does not stop working, and we wake feeling exhausted. This system also believes that the second best choice, if we cannot face north, is to face east. Chinese practitioners of Feng Shui believe that east is the best direction to face when sleeping, and when we face west during sleep, the conscious mind stays busy and we can't fully rest.

Now, some studies suggest those who sleep with their heads facing east have less REM sleep (dream state), while those who face north have more REM sleep. So, for someone who feels they dream too much—which is not restful, because we restore our bodies during non-REM sleep—or for anyone prone to nightmares, it would be

K.W. PETERS

worth experimenting with facing east while sleeping, to see if that reduced excessive dreaming.

One reference I found while researching this subject offered a reasonable solution to the quandary. It pointed out those living in the Northern hemisphere should face north when sleeping, and those living in the Southern hemisphere should face south; this would explain the opposing viewpoints of the Eastern and Western traditions.

Given the conflicting information on this topic, I was tempted to simply leave this material out of the book. However, I do believe there is some importance to the direction we face while we sleep, and it may be the missing piece of the sleeping puzzle for some people (who have tried everything else, to no avail). The obvious thing to do here is to experiment.

If you have ongoing sleeping problems, or wake fatigued and devoid of energy, try to sleep facing another direction for a few days, and see if that makes a difference. After all, given the critical importance of getting regular, good quality sleep, anything that could help attain this, is worth considering.

BEDDING AND SLEEPWEAR

Given that the body detoxifies through the skin at night, it is important to sleep with fabrics that breathe. Therefore, it is recommended one use mattresses made of natural materials (such as cotton futons), and that all bedding and sleepwear be made of natural fabrics.

Using polyester and other synthetic fibers in nighttime clothing, bedding, and mattresses, is like sleeping in a plastic bag. Our body is then forced to consume foul air, filled with its own off-gassed toxins—causing us to reabsorb those toxins.

As well, static electricity fields are created by ions released from synthetic materials in the home, and can build up enough of a charge to make one feel unwell. This can be avoided by also using natural fabrics for carpets, couches, curtains, pillows, etc.

There is another important—if somewhat disgusting—fact to be aware of. After 5 years (or so) of use, up to 50% of the weight of a pillow, or mattress, is comprised of dust mites, and dust mite excrement. Breathing this in is linked to asthma, and other breathing problems, which can also interfere with a good night's sleep.

This is one reason why I like cotton futons—they can easily, and inexpensively, be replaced every 5 years or so. Pillows should be replaced at least every 3 years, since your face is bouncing around on it every night, potentially creating small dust clouds for you to inhale.

Because we detoxify at night, it is also important we have as much clean, fresh air as possible, therefore, whenever it is reasonable, one should keep a window open while sleeping.

TOXIC MATTRESSES

Most new, commercial mattresses produce toxins as they gas-off, and every time you shift positions in your bed, you release volatile organic compounds (VOCs) from the mattress into your breathing space. This occurs because most mattresses are made of petroleum-based polyurethane foam, which release VOCs. As well, some of the adhesives used to hold mattresses together contain, and release, formaldehyde.

On top of that, all mattresses (including foam) are required by law to have flame retardants applied to them. However, mattress companies are not very forthcoming on what flame-retardants they are currently using—though most likely they are using flame retardant materials such as modacrylic fiber (that contains the carcinogenic heavy metal antimony), and PBDE's (polybrominated diphenyl ethers).

Lest you think "Memory Foam" mattresses may be a better choice, they were lab tested by Walter Bader—while doing research for his book "Toxic Bedrooms"—and found to emit 61 chemicals, including the carcinogens benzene, and naphthalene.

K. W. PETERS

Infants face a higher risk from toxic mattresses because they are less able to process toxins, and they spend more time sleeping than adults. One study of new and used crib mattresses detected VOCs in all the mattress samples (though the levels of VOCs emitted from newer mattresses were higher than levels emitted from used ones). The study also showed polyurethane foam mattresses released a greater number of VOCs than did those made of polyester foam.

Older mattresses, which have been around a few years, have outgassed most of the toxic chemicals, and mattresses made before 2007, generally, have not have been contaminated with PBDEs (flame- retardants).

However, aside from the ick-factor of buying a used bed, we have to take into account the build-up of dust mites, which occurs in old mattresses. So, when buying a second hand mattress, try to ensure the mattress was seldom used (such as one from a guest room). And, keep in mind, while older mattresses may be done gassing off after a few years, the same does not hold true for foam mattresses since, as foam degrades, it releases even more PBDEs than when it is new.

The best solution here is to purchase organic mattresses made with natural latex, or old style futons made exclusively from cotton. Most futons for sale these days have a foam core, and covers that have flame-retardants applied, so you will have to do some research to ensure you have the safest bed possible.

One good mattress choice is available at www.intellibed.com. They use an inert, silica-coated, mineral-based fire retardant. This type of fire retardant is not bio-available through any contact, and is not broken down through body heat, pressure, or liquid—it is only activated when the mattress is on fire.

SEROTONIN

Serotonin is one of our two main calming neurotransmitters (the other being GABA). If you lay in bed at night with your brain racing, worrying about the day and unable to shut down, this indicates you are deficient in serotonin. Another symptom of serotonin deficiency occurs when you twitch just as you are about to fall asleep. This feels like a slight, spastic jerk that brings you back to wakefulness, with the sense that you had just been falling.

For this common form of sleep disorder, the approach is two-fold: first we set the body up to increase its serotonin levels (thus shutting down the "rooftop chatter"), then we prime the pineal pump with a little melatonin.

Now, melatonin produces some serotonin, and vice-versa, so ideally we are using a bit of both instead of too much of one. That being said, if one cannot take melatonin (for example if it causes too much dreaming, or if the party in question is an adolescent), then just increasing serotonin may produce enough melatonin to do the job.

The primary serotonin precursors generally used are L-theanine, 5-HTP, tryptophan, or vitamin B-3 (as niacinamide, intermediate release flush-free niacin, or regular flushing niacin for those who can tolerate it).

Of these options, L-theanine (an amino acid derived from green tea) is my favorite, since it is safe enough to be used by children, and pregnant or nursing women. It also does not interact with other medications, unlike 5-HTP or tryptophan, which should not be taken by those using anti-depressants. In fact, L-theanine is so effective, in Japan it is used to treat children with attention deficit hyperactivity disorder (ADHD). To aid in sleeping, one usually takes from 250 mg to 500 mg of L-theanine, about 15 to 20 minutes before bed.

A little trial and error may be necessary to find which substance—and what dosage—work best for you. Whichever substance you find the most effective, the end result is roughly the same: the brain quiets down and moves into an alpha-wave state. This state is attained during meditation, and occurs just prior to entering the dream-state, known scientifically as theta-wave activity. From the dream state, we ideally descend to the delta-wave state, which is deep sleep. Here no

K.W. PETERS

dream activity occurs and the body repairs and restores itself; this is the most critical area of sleep required to ensure good health.

As we return to consciousness, we pass from delta, back through theta to alpha, and finally come to the beta wave state, which is alert wakefulness. This pattern illustrates why we generally only remember the dreams we have before waking.

If a serotonin booster does not help, you might try using GABA (our other main inhibitory neurotransmitter). Usually 250 to 500 mg is taken shortly before bed, while those who have serious daytime anxiety will use that much three times daily. Recently, a clinically researched GABA has entered the market. PharmaGABA is naturally derived, and appears to work at a lower dose (and more effectively) than generic GABA products (which are usually synthetic).

Some people may find that both serotonin boosters and GABA are required to effect full relaxation.

HOW TO USE MELATONIN

For recommended dosage levels of melatonin (based on your age), please see the chapter on that subject. For most people, one to three milligrams is usually sufficient, especially if combined with a serotonin booster.

So, first we ingest one or more of these serotonin producing substances (and possibly some GABA), about 15 to 20 minutes before retiring, in order to prepare the brain for sleep. Then we take our melatonin sublingually, 5 or 10 minutes before shutting off the light. We do this because light dissipates melatonin: if we take it too early, exposure to light will just dissolve it out of the bloodstream.

This tendency of melatonin to dissipate is also the reason you must sleep in a room that is as dark as possible. (Street light shining in through bedroom windows is one of the main causes of sleep disorders in city dwellers.) If you have to get up at night to use the washroom, try to use as little light as possible.

A small night light can be helpful here, since weak light will not be as disruptive to melatonin levels (nor will red light, since it does not affect melatonin at all). However, if you turn the lights on fully, you may find it difficult to get back to sleep again, as most of your melatonin will have dissipated. At this point more sedative agents (like L-Theanine) can be ingested, but, if dawn is approaching, more melatonin may leave you groggy when you waken.

Waking up in the middle of the night can be related to adrenal gland exhaustion. This problem more often strikes those in their later years, when the adrenals have been run down by years of stress and stimulants (even as simple as too much sugar and/or coffee). For women undergoing menopause, hot flashes can make sleeping even more difficult. Taking an adrenal rebuilding formula can, over time, help with the sleep disorder, and aid in balancing the sex hormones—in turn helping to alleviate the hot flashes. Sage pills (such as "Menopause" from A. Vogel) can also help women who have hot flashes.

VITAMIN D AND INSOMNIA

Sleep disorders have become epidemic throughout the world over the last 40 years. It is during this timeframe that we also find a large portion of the population spending the majority of their lives indoors. This has led to a worldwide epidemic of vitamin D deficiency (for example, more than 80% of people in India and Saudi Arabia are vitamin D deficient).

I have covered vitamin D extensively in my blogs (as well as in Volume One of Health Secrets, and in a free E-book on the subject—available at www.nutristart.com), but here I will touch on the link between vitamin D deficiency and insomnia.

In 2012, a group of scientists hypothesized that because "vitamin D plays an important role in the brainstem control of sleep, the prevalence of vitamin D deficiency is the cause of the current epidemic of sleep disorders". The validity of their thesis was supported by the fact there are vitamin D receptors in many parts of the brain—including "areas that are considered to play a role in the initiation and maintenance of sleep".

These researchers performed a two-year study, supplementing vitamin D to 1500 patients with neurological complaints, who also had sleep disorders. Results indicated most of the patients "had improvement in neurologic symptoms and sleep but only through maintaining a narrow range of 25(OH) vitamin D3 blood levels of 60-80 ng/ml".

The surprising thing here was the specific window of effectiveness: blood levels of 60-80 ng/ml. Now, I state in my earlier material that the ideal blood level of vitamin D is around 50 ng/ml—this being based on information from The Vitamin D Council, and from the world's foremost expert on vitamin D, Dr. Michael Holick.

Yet, here they discovered that "the sleep difficulties produced by vitamin D levels below 50 ng/ml return, in the same form, as the level goes over 80 ng/ml, suggesting a narrower range of 'normal' vitamin D levels for sleep than those published for bone health". This implies those with chronic insomnia may need to fine-tune their blood levels of vitamin D, in order to improve their sleep patterns. This can be accomplished with vitamin D testing—available on-line, or through a doctor.

Another interesting discovery from this study, was that vitamin D2 (ergocalciferol, found in prescription vitamin D products, some supplements, and fortifying some foods), prevented normal sleep in most patients. This does not surprise me, as I have already covered the counterproductive nature of vitamin D2 in my blogs, and books, on the subject.

OTHER OPTIONS

For some people a sleep aid can be as simple as taking a combination of the herbs valerian and lemon balm—proven effective in European studies. Usually the herbal approach works best for simple stress that does not include much exposure to electromagnetic pollution.

Other sedative herbs, with a long historical track record for efficiency, include skullcap (used also for meditation, as it quiets an agitated brain), hops (which also have estrogenic properties, helpful during menopause), and passionflower (especially good for daytime anxiety). All these herbs (along with the serotonin precursors discussed) can also be used during the daytime as stress-reducers, and anti-anxiety agents. (Though, be sure you are familiar with the effects before driving, or operating machinery.)

For children, and hypersensitive adults, with sleeping problems, look to homeopathic remedies, such as Hyland's Calms Forte, or Chamomilla (a homeopathic version of the herb chamomile), both of which can be safely used by anyone, including infants.

Homeopathics work as a catalyst for the body, without having a direct mechanical effect (unlike the previous substances we discussed). This also makes them safe for people who are on medications (such as anti-depressants, which forbid the use of 5-HTP and GABA), since there are no interactions between homeopathics and pharmaceuticals.

Finally, a couple of considerations derived from Chinese medicine. Practitioners of this modality suggest that reading non-fiction before bed stimulates the mind too much (by overworking the spleen meridian), but reading fiction does not have this effect. So, I keep my book-learning confined to the day and early evening, and always have a comfortable piece of fiction by my bedside.

Another recommendation found in Chinese medicine, based on the principles of Feng Shui, is to ensure you can see the bedroom door from your bed. This allows your instinctive brain to relax, knowing no one can sneak up on you while you sleep.

PART TWO

RADIATION AND XENOESTROGENS

CHAPTER ONE

RADIATION

The subject of radiation was a hot topic in 2011, when the Fukushima nuclear power plant (in Japan) was destroyed by a tsunami. However, as time went on, the Western media stopped discussing it, and soon people put it to the back of their minds.

THE GOVERNMENT WON'T PROTECT YOU

At that time, the Canadian and American governments betrayed their citizens by failing to track increasing levels of radiation in rainwater and food, and by not warning the most sensitive among us to take precautions. Those in most danger included pregnant women (specifically their unborn), those about to become pregnant, and the immune-compromised.

Following the Fukushima meltdown, the Environmental Protection Agency (EPA) pulled 8 of its 18 radiation monitors in California, Oregon, and Washington State, because the monitors were recording readings which seemed too high (www.washingtonsblog.com). Six months after the meltdown, American and Canadian authorities virtually stopped monitoring airborne radiation.

Shortly after the Fukushima disaster, journalist Alex Roslin (Georgia Straight magazine) reported that a Health Canada monitoring station in Sidney, B.C., had detected radioactive iodine-131 up to 300 times more than normal background levels. Meanwhile, Health Canada was declaring on its website that the quantities of radiation reaching Canada did not pose any health risk to Canadians.

Here on the west coast of B.C., one company stopped harvesting bladderwrack (a seaweed that floats near the top of the ocean), due to the high amount of radiation it picked up from rainwater, following the disaster. During this time, an acquaintance of mine was contacted by a concerned friend who lived in South Korea. There, the news programs were showing the west coast of B.C. as a danger zone for radiation.

Where was our government in all of this? Protecting business, which appears to be the main motivation for Western democracy these days. As well, there is no doubt that the nuclear industry, poised for resurgence as an alternative to fossil fuels, was putting a reverse spin on the information—minimizing the dangers.

Canada sells nuclear reactors around the world, and this industry was readying for a comeback—now able to ride the "green" train, promoting nuclear fuel as a cleaner substitute for coal, and petrochemicals. The Japanese meltdown derailed that train, so their best option was to wait quietly until people forgot about it. Which is what occurred.

We are still receiving conflicting information about the amount, and dangers of, radiation we are receiving from Japan here in North America. Something to be concerned about, since Fukushima is still dumping huge amounts of radioactive water into the Pacific Ocean. (Last estimate is 300 tons, daily, since 2011.)

Therefore, it behooves us to know as much as possible about ways to aid the body in coping with the radiation that will keep building up in our bodies, over time. As well, a good chance of other nuclear emergencies occurring exists, especially since there are many old-model nuclear reactors in North America—many on, or close to, fault lines.

In 2014, President Obama approved raising the permissible levels of nuclear radiation in drinking water and soil, allowing guidelines "many times more lax than anything EPA has ever before accepted". These guides govern evacuations, shelter-in-place orders, food restrictions, and other actions, following a wide range of "radiological emergencies". Such potential future events include nuclear-reactor meltdowns, dirty-bomb attacks, or other unexpected releases of radiation.

Radiation is the detrimental "gift that keeps on giving", since all of the radiation that has entered the environment remains there—for a very long time. Instead, it will move up the food chain, concentrating in fish, dairy foods, animal flesh, and ultimately, in our bodies.

SYMPTOMS OF RADIATION EXPOSURE

There are many harmful effects of radiation, but since the damage can build slowly, many of them go unnoticed. Over time, a low level of radiation exposure can lead to major digestive imbalances, blood alterations, and destruction of tissue and organ systems at a cellular level. Low-level symptoms can include fatigue, headaches, nausea, scalp issues, and dry/itchy skin. As things get worse, due either to long-term build-up, or extreme short-term exposure, symptoms can include attention disorders, brain damage, memory problems, mood changes, and reduced cognitive and psychomotor abilities.

Radiation has an effect on the circulatory system, reducing blood lymphocytes, which in turn can lead to higher incidence of bodily infections. Mild radiation poisoning causes flu-like symptoms, and can increase your future risk of developing cancers of the blood (leukemia and lymphoma). Long-term radiation exposure can affect the reproductive system, leading to birth defects, infertility, and stillbirths.

FEAR

Discussing radiation is a loaded subject, since such discussions can easily turn into fear mongering. So, on the one hand, we have silence from the government, and conventional media, and on the other, we have internet hysteria. The long-lasting damage to individuals caught up in the Chernobyl meltdown (1986) was a result of fear and stress, more than actual radiation damage—not counting infants and children.

In his book, "Healing with Whole Foods", Paul Pitchford noted that, following the Chernobyl meltdown, many health-inclined people in North America made themselves sick by overeating miso and seaweed, along with copious amounts of detoxifying green foods—much sicker than they would have gotten from the small amount of radiation issuing from Chernobyl. (However, that was a much smaller event than Fukushima.)

Such related hysteria followed the Japanese situation. Health food stores could not keep seaweed and iodine products in stock. People were angry at the lack of stock (though who could have prepared for this?), fearful from receiving conflicting information (conventional news media vs internet), and generally over-stressed.

These kind of emotions (when they run wild) do not allow us to think clearly, and add stress, burdening the adrenal glands. The further stress on the adrenals may cause an overload, if these glands are already overworked, due to coping with radiation. Unfortunately, given the human tendency to swing from one extreme to another, hysteria gave way to apathy and now (due in part to the media sweeping it under the rug), nobody talks about it. Thus, few people are incorporating anti-radiation elements into their health regimes anymore.

A BALANCED APPROACH

In the chapters concerning radiation, I will present the best long-term solutions to dealing with an environment that, from now forward, will likely contain dangerous amounts of radiation. Radiation, like many modern invisible agents working towards our demise, is defined as a "cumulative carcinogen" (chlorine being another example). Essentially, this means it is not a question of how much radiation you absorbed *today* (unless you are next door to a meltdown)—the concern is the amount accumulated over decades (which leads to an increase in your overall cancer risk).

Fortunately, there are foods, supplements, and techniques that pull radiation out of our bodies, lessening the total load, and offering us protection. These approaches should now become part of your lifestyle—and that of your children, and their children. I also suggest avoiding X-rays and CT scans, as much as possible; the extra radiation load is no longer going to be as "safe" as it used to be.

IT'S NOT THE FIRST TIME

The reality is, we already have large amounts of radiation in our environment from decades of above-ground nuclear testing—courtesy of all the major superpowers in the world. Even after the U.S. ceased above-ground testing (and turned to below-ground testing), Russia, China, France, and North Korea, were all still testing above-ground. One source maintained that over 2,000 various types of atomic bombs were tested above-ground during this time, with half of them being American tests done in North America, or in the Pacific Ocean.

The current Japanese situation is merely topping up the pre-existing radiation in our environment. Therefore, the anti-radiation protocols that follow should be considered suggestions for long-term use, not just something for this latest crisis.

Since radiation poisoning is generally based on lifetime exposure, we must include what we accumulate from medical and dental x-rays, exposure from flying, and what we acquire from foods that store radiation (bananas, brazil nuts, dairy products, fish and meat). Tobacco will add considerably to the radiation load of smokers, since it both pulls radiation from the environment, and is commonly grown with phosphate fertilizers that contain radioactive polonium-210.

A new source of airborne radiation is resulting from increased frequency of wild fires in North America and around the world. As radiation is taken up from the soil into plants, a fair amount of it is sequestered in trees and, during forest fires, released into the atmosphere with smoke. It has been determined that recent forest fires around Chernobyl have released large amounts of radiation into the atmosphere over Eastern Europe. Therefore, those who are concerned should consider wearing facemasks (N95 type), when wildfire smoke is present in their environment.

POTASSIUM IODIDE

Most people have heard about the protective benefits of iodine, following exposure to nuclear radiation. So, let's have a closer look at that subject, clarify some of the issues surrounding the initial hysterical consumer demand for iodine, and distinguish between iodine and potassium iodide.

Firstly, we need to understand that most people are deficient in iodine, and, because your body cannot distinguish between iodine the mineral and radioactive iodine, it will absorb whichever is present first. Therefore, if airborne radiation passes over you, or you eat food contaminated with radioactive iodine, your body will easily absorb that radioactive iodine into the thyroid gland. That is, unless your thyroid gland is already full of natural iodine, in which case radioactive iodine can find no purchase there.

If you have not been consuming iodine on a regular basis, and a radioactive cloud approaches your vicinity, you should take large doses of iodine (in the form of potassium iodide), in order to prevent the thyroid gland from absorbing radioactive iodine.

There is much confusion about the distinction between iodine and potassium iodide. Seaweed products (food or pills) provide iodine, which—after being converted by the body into iodide—will saturate and protect the thyroid (since the thyroid only uptakes iodine in this form). However, this takes much longer to do than directly ingesting potassium iodide as a supplement.

Potassium iodide has a direct affinity for the thyroid gland, and will immediately lodge there, blocking the uptake of radioactive iodine. However, radioactive iodine, while it is the most abundant, is only one of the radioactive elements. Although iodide will protect the thyroid, it will not stop radiation uptake in other areas of the body, nor will it protect against other forms of radiation (which will be addressed shortly), and it will not aid in removal of radiation from the body.

One of the few potassium iodide products approved by the FDA, in case of nuclear emergency, is Thyrosafe (www.thyrosafe.com). Following the Fukushima disaster, people were clamoring for this, and related products, based mostly on internet pseudo-news, but the majority were, for the most part, unaware of the risk-to-benefit ratio of these types of products.

Because the recommended dose is 130 mg for an adult—providing 100 mg of elemental iodide—the product is dangerous to use, outside of a full-scale nuclear meltdown in your vicinity. The children's dose is 65 mg for 3 to 18 year olds, 32 mg for 1 month to 3 years old, and 16 mg for under-one-month old. Fortunately, radioactive iodine has a half-life of 8 days (further reducing by half every 8 days), so these strong potassium iodide products need only be used for a short period—generally, 3 days is suggested.

IF YOU LIVE NEAR A NUCLEAR PLANT

These strong potassium iodide products are issued to people who live near nuclear power plants (to be used in case of meltdown). But, for those who live anywhere in the vicinity of a nuclear power plant, it is a good idea to keep some on hand.

I live on the West Coast of B.C., and in nearby Washington State there is an older model (functioning) nuclear power plant—along with stored nuclear waste. Since the West Coast is considered a "red zone" for earthquake potential, and the reactor in question is situated near a fault line, it is logical for those who live in its vicinity to consider adding Thyrosafe (or a similar product) to their earthquake kits. However, when considering the amount of radiation the wind may carry over from Japan (or from any meltdown that is far away), a product like Thyrosafe is overkill, and the risk of iodine overdose outweighs any protective benefits offered.

Currently, most authorities suggest that taking slightly more iodine than the RDI (150 mcg for an adult) is sufficient protection against what radiation we might receive from Japan. So, acquiring from 150 mcg of iodine (which can be found in most multivitamins), up to 300 mcg (which can be gained by an additional iodine supplement, or some seaweed), should be enough to protect our thyroids, in this case.

Potassium iodide only protects the thyroid from up-taking radioactive iodine, but will do so quickly. Regular iodine confers broader protection, and will also protect the thyroid (though it takes longer to reach that gland). This delay in absorption occurs because there are iodine receptors throughout the body, and iodine will occupy all these sites on its way to the thyroid. So, during a meltdown, we only want potassium iodide, but generally, we want a good consistent intake of iodine, to protect us now, and in the future.

SEAWEED AND IODINE

A gram (1000 mg) of kelp (dried or in tablet) provides roughly between 500 and 1000 mcg (0.5 to 1 mg) of iodine, which is more than enough, based on Western standards. I believe, however, in taking higher levels of iodine than are commonly recommended by Western medicine. My belief is based, in part, on the Japanese average daily intake of iodine—far higher than in the West. This high intake aids in protecting them against many diseases, and keeps their thyroids well-saturated with iodine. Having their thyroids pre-saturated with iodine, was certainly lifesaving for those living close to

Fukushima when the meltdown occurred. (And we might say the same about those who survived Hiroshima and Nagasaki.)

Since the Japanese acquire from 1 to 3 mg of iodine daily—mostly from eating seaweed—I feel we can safely take much more than the RDI (150 mcg). Though, when taking iodine as an isolated nutrient (in supplement form), remember that almost all nutrients require secondary nutrients for their assimilation. In the case of iodine, it most importantly requires extra selenium and tin (a trace mineral required in small amounts).

When eating seaweed, all the cofactors are present (as it is a whole food). However, when taking supplemental iodine at higher doses (milligrams rather than micrograms), I suggest adding a selenium supplement (if not taking a multivitamin), and using trace mineral drops (such as "Concentrace").

STAY INFORMED

Most of the damage following the Chernobyl crisis occurred in the decades that followed, with increased cancer rates in the surrounding areas and countries. With Fukushima, the story is no longer "news", though the plant in question is still spewing radioactivity into the ocean.

Apart from radioactive iodine (which has a short half-life), other radioactive material is just going to keep circulating, settling into the environment, and moving up the food chain. Therefore, I strongly suggest continuing to follow information on the Japanese nuclear crisis, because our government officials are not going to keep us up to date. And, while most of the contamination is currently entering the ocean, another severe earthquake could see that radiation airborne again, further worsening our dangers.

In fact, the huge amounts of radiation entering the Pacific Ocean (from Fukushima), may be responsible for strange occurrences happening, not long ago, on our shores. Have a look at these related news stories:

- CBS: "Mysterious whale deaths" in California under investigation—Scientists perplexed—"Continues trend of whales washing ashore"—Animals sick, starving, emaciated, too weak to swim, hemorrhaging. (April 29, 2015)

- ENENews: Dead sea creatures "covering the sand with a sea of red" on California beach; Witnesses: "Bazillions of crab-like things washed ashore...I've never seen these before, it's incredible." (March 23, 2015)

- CBS: Officials alarmed as several types of marine mammals begin washing up in California—"Now entire coast is being affected."—"Whole population getting hit hard... a real shock to us."—"Animals of all ages sick, not only newborns." (February 2, 2015)

- Guardian: Pacific Ocean "turning into a desert" off California—Experts: "Entire generation of baby sea lions is dying."; "It's incredible, it's so unusual and there's no good explanation for it."; "Expect same thing to happen again next year—Carts filled with emaciated dead bodies." (May 17, 2015)

- ABC: "Mysterious surge" in sick marine mammals all along California coast—Infested with parasites, extremely emaciated; "Very seriously ill...in very bad shape"—Experts: "We're extremely concerned right now—Deaths up 1,500% at rescue facility." (Jan 13, 2015)

It is not my desire to add to the propagation of fear, nor do I wish to minimize the problem by suggesting the relatively small amounts of radiation we receive does not impact our health. All of the radiation absorbed from rain, watersheds, and our foods—especially Pacific fish, dairy products and meats—cause free radical damage throughout the body.

Since we are constantly exposed to radiation (from medical and dental treatments, the remains of above-ground nuclear testing, and from nuclear accidents), the next two chapters are designed to empower you with knowledge needed to stay safe year-round. Do not

K. W. PETERS

wait until faced with the next nuclear disaster to implement the recommendations to follow (believe me, Fukushima is not the last one we will see). Now let's move from exploring the problem, to finding solutions that protect us, and our loved ones.

RADIOPROTECTIVE FOODS

"All French citizens were warned against consuming rainwater, leafy greens, and all milk derived products (including from goats and sheep, as well as cows), due to radioactive fallout contamination in Europe. The U.S. and Canadian governments still claim that all of the above foods are safe in North America, even for infants and pregnant women; unfortunately the reality is that the level of radioactive fallout present here is 8 to 10 times greater that of France and the rest of Europe."

This material was taken from a website (www.enenews.com) designed to keep us updated on radiation status in the world. I was recommending this site (in my original draft), but as of now (2019) is has been removed from the web. (Insert conspiracy theory here.) Enenews.com, offered material conventional media does not seem interesting in reporting—or are not allowed to report. Given General Electric owns countless media outlets, and is in partnership with producers of nuclear technology, it is not a great leap to assume they might not want information broadcast which could impede the development of their nuclear business. And, since the google search engine has become a tool for conventional business interests, it is no surprise to find such sites shut down, most likely for providing "fake news". Nonetheless, the archives for this website are available at www. healfukushima.org, along with current information on Fukushima.

CHOOSING SAFE FOODS

What we know now is the entire Northern Hemisphere, and the Pacific Ocean, received the bulk of the radiation spewing out of the damaged Fukushima reactor—with the areas worst hit being Japan, and the Pacific Rim countries. Therefore, food grown in these areas will be the most contaminated, especially the Pacific coastal areas.

Though the Fukushima plant was eventually contained, and the winds and rain stopped carrying radiation over here, we still have to live with the residue that is in the soil. This radiation will move up the food chain, through grass and plants, into meat and dairy products.

Obviously, fish harvested from around Japan are already too con-taminated to eat. And, given the radioactive water dumped daily into the ocean since 2011, it is only a matter of time until most fish in the Pacific Ocean end up somewhat contaminated—with the largest, longest-living fish, carrying the most radiation.

There has been little fallout in the Southern Hemisphere, but this area was also affected by the huge amount of radiation dumped into the Pacific Ocean. It did not take long for Australia to find fish con-taminated with radiation, in their waters.

Currently, the safest areas of origin for food that is uncontami-nated are Africa, Central America (but not Mexican food from their Pacific Coast), and South America. Unfortunately, these are also areas with little in the way of environmental protection agencies. Therefore, food from these areas may be more contaminated with pesticides than North American produce. So essentially it is a case of "pick your poison".

The best we can do is focus on organic foods, to reduce other contaminants, and try to break even to some degree. Europe, while receiving some of the fallout, is still a better choice for animal foods than North America, and for North American animal foods, focus on those produced on the East Coast first, and then the central areas next. Plant-based foods are not as much of a concern, since they are lower on the food chain.

Some authorities have suggested freezing fish and milk (and milk products) for two weeks before consuming. This allows time for radioactive iodine to decay to the point of not being dangerous (though it does not address the other radioactive elements). However, this approach should only be necessary during a nuclear crisis—such as the beginning of the Fukushima meltdown, when radiation was carried in the wind and rain, over to the West Coast. Since radioactive iodine has a short half-life, this approach is not of value right now.

RADIOPROTECTIVE FOODS

First, and foremost, eat more seaweed. While many in the West have never acquired a taste for this food (outside of sushi), it is a superior food in many ways. For example, Chinese medicine uses seaweed to treat tumors, and growths in the body. But, for our purposes, the extremely high level of iodine found in seaweed protects the thyroid, while high amounts of other minerals, helps protect the rest of the body from radiation damage.

Brown seaweeds, including alaria, kelp, kombu, bladderwrack, and wakame, are also high in algin, which will actually pull radiation from the body. (Algin, as an isolate, is sometimes found in supplements, listed as "sodium alginate".) For those not keen on seaweed, nori (used to wrap sushi), and dulse, are two of the tastier seaweeds, and easy to add to soups, salads, or grains.

Now, we do have to try to determine the location the seaweed was harvested from, since obviously we do not want Japanese seaweed. Nor do we want any harvested from the Pacific Rim countries, as seaweed can pick up and store radiation. Atlantic dulse is a good choice, as it is harvested from the East Coast.

K.W. PETERS

ALKALINE DIET AND RADIATION

Some of the damage caused by radiation is due to it creating a high level of acidity in the body. Therefore, all alkalizing foods are protective, especially organic vegetables, which are rich in minerals. Organic food contains the full range of trace minerals, whereas agribusiness vegetables are not only lacking in minerals—due to topsoil erosion and use of synthetic fertilizers—but also contain high amounts of pesticide residue, which is highly acidic to the body.

As an aside, the acid/alkaline theory is not based on any actual change in the pH of blood—if your pH did change, you would simply die. This is the reason many doctors do not believe it is a valid theory. In fact, the theory is based on the tendency of the body to neutralize acidic foods (and substances) by pulling minerals out of the body, in order to maintain the ideal pH of blood necessary for life. Since minerals are alkalizing, the more we lose from our bodies and bones over time, the weaker and more acidic our systems become. Acidity is also related to inflammation, and inflammation is, in turn, related to a host of diseases.

By now, most of us know which foods are acidifying (sugars, refined carbs, fruit juices, "bad" fats, excessive meat, excessive refined salt, etc.), and which foods are alkalizing (whole vegetables, dark leafy green vegetables, essential fatty acids, berries, whole grains, natural salts, lean proteins, sprouted and fermented foods, etc.). It is also important to keep up a good intake of filtered, or spring, water, when the body is coping with any additional toxic burden.

MISO

Followers of Macrobiotics—a Japanese dietary philosophy based on Zen Buddhism—maintain that, after the bombing of Hiroshima and Nagasaki, residents not directly affected by the blast, who consumed brown rice and miso, did not suffer as much from the effects of radiation sickness, as did those who were eating a modern diet.

Miso is a traditional Japanese paste (usually used to make soup) made from fermented soybeans and rice, and is one of the few unpasteurized foods available in modern times. In Japan, and among health food aficionados, miso is believed to provide health-promoting benefits, including reducing fatigue, regulating intestinal functions, aiding digestion, protecting against gastric ulcers, lowering cholesterol and blood pressure, and preventing lifestyle diseases like cancer.

Recently, a series of mice studies done in Japan confirmed the anecdotal information regarding miso preventing radiation sickness. There was one caveat though: "However, this phenomenon was not observed when miso was given on 0, 1, or 2 days after irradiation. So it was concluded that a certain concentration of the effective substance(s) must exist in the blood before exposure." (1)

In other words, you need to have built-up the benefits of miso before it can protect you from dramatic radiation exposure, such as during a nuclear crisis. Therefore, now is the time to add this superior food to your diet, for long term protection.

When making miso soup, the important thing to remember is not to boil it. Miso is added to hot water after boiling ceases, in order not to destroy the live enzymes it contains. Since most soybeans are genetically modified these days, always be sure to purchase a miso made from organic soybeans. For those allergic to soy, there is now miso made from other types of beans, although we cannot yet be sure that these alternative miso products will have the same radio-protective effects as miso made from soybeans.

We can also assume that, as part of their traditional diet, the Japanese who coped well with nuclear fallout, also consumed high amounts of brown rice, green tea (extremely high in antioxidants), and, of course, seaweed. These foods are all very alkalizing so much of their benefit may simply come from neutralizing the high acidity caused by radiation exposure.

SULFUR FOODS

Some other foods have a particular ability to help protect the body from radiation, and to help flush it out before it can do too much damage. These especially include the sulfur-containing foods (such as cabbage, broccoli, Brussels sprouts, cauliflower, kale, and eggs) since sulfur helps the body produce the powerful antioxidant glutathione.

Glutathione is the single most important antioxidant that we require, and is necessary for the body to detoxify properly. This is due to glutathione being the only key antioxidant that acts inside the cell—all other antioxidants work outside the cell membranes. Glutathione is therefore essential for protecting cellular DNA from oxidative damage caused by free radicals.

The above-mentioned cruciferous vegetables should usually be cooked before eating, since when consumed raw they can inhibit iodine uptake by the thyroid gland.

Other foods rich in sulfur include members of the onion and garlic family, including chives, leeks, shallots, and scallions. In fact, garlic extracts have been studied for their radioprotective function, and were found to protect red blood cells from radiation damage, and to prevent radiation damage to chromosomes in the bone marrow cells, via glutathione production. (2)

Beans are also sulfur-containing and, in moderation, can be an alkalizing source of protein in the diet. For those who choose to reduce or avoid using animal proteins, beans are an important food to add to the diet. However, you should ideally choose your beans based on your blood type, for optimal digestion, and health benefits.

OTHER PROTECTIVE FOODS

Apples

Apples are high in the fiber pectin, which binds and removes radiation from the body. They are also particularly high in calcium d-glucarate—a natural substance with powerful detoxification properties. Grapefruit is also high in both pectin and calcium d-glucarate. Just make sure your apples, or grapefruits, are organic—especially since non-organic versions of these fruits are notoriously high in pesticides.

Beets

Red beets can aid the body in rebuilding damaged hemoglobin—the primary component of red blood cells, broken down by exposure to radiation. In animal studies, beets have been shown to absorb and detoxify radioactive isotopes. (3)

Buckwheat

Buckwheat is rich in rutin, a bioflavonoid that protects against radiation damage. Rutin strengthens the capillary walls, and can reduce hemorrhaging caused by x-rays. Animal studies have shown rutin dramatically reduces death rates caused by excessive radiation exposure, mostly through protecting the gastrointestinal tract, and bone marrow. Protection was noted to begin at 10 mg of rutin per kilo of body weight, though the study went as high as 40 mg per kilo. Rutin is available as an inexpensive supplement, commonly used to treat hemorrhoids, and varicose veins. (4)

Flaxseed

A mouse study, done at the University of Pennsylvania, discovered that flaxseed powerfully protects lungs from radiation damage. They found this seed protected tissue and organs most effectively when taken before exposure to radiation, but it also reduced damage when taken after exposure.

Flaxseed contains strong antioxidants in the form of lignans, which can safely remove certain chemical pollutants from the body. And, of course, flax oil, contained in the seeds, is high in omega 3 fatty acids, which serve as an anti-inflammatory, and protect cell membranes from rupturing. Both these mechanisms are helpful when coping with radiation damage.

The mice in this study were fed a diet containing 10% flaxseeds, which they received either 3 weeks before having their thorax X-rayed, or at 2, 4, or 6 weeks after being exposed to radiation. A control group had the same diet, and the same radiation exposure, but were given no flax seeds.

At the end of 4 months, 70 to 80 percent of the irradiated mice fed flaxseeds had survived, compared to only 40% of the control group that did not receive flaxseeds. The study concluded that, "...dietary flaxseed may be clinically useful as an agent to increase the therapeutic index of thoracic X-ray radiation therapy by increasing the radiation tolerance of lung tissues". (5)

Ginger

Ginger extract has shown to boost glutathione activity, and reduce lipid peroxidation, by scavenging free radicals immediately following exposure to lethal radiation doses. This means it both reduces the cellular damage radiation causes, and helps the body detoxify radiation that is absorbed.

However, the study showing ginger protecting mice against radiation damage, supplied ginger extract to the rodents before exposing them to gamma radiation. Ginger did indeed reduce symptoms of radiation poisoning, and prevented ensuing gastrointestinal and bone marrow related deaths. But, providing ginger after exposing the mice to lethal radiation, provided little benefit—so don't wait to add ginger to your diet. (6)

Ginger is a wonderful spice, serving as a digestive and circulatory aid, a powerful anti-inflammatory, and helping the body cope with a variety of toxins. It can be added to food (freshly grated being superior to powdered), eaten as gingered candy, or drunk as a beverage— as herbal tea, or even as a natural ginger ale (with at least 5% ginger).

Green Tea

Green tea is a powerful antioxidant, protecting against general free radical damage, and specifically protecting against side effects from gamma radiation. Green tea has many health benefits, most of which are based on drinking 3 to 5 cups daily.

Those who are not fond of green tea as a beverage can purchase it as a liquid concentrate, or in capsule form, in order to consume enough to be protective. However, green tea supplements should be as close as possible to the whole plant, since even removing the caffeine from green tea reduces its benefits: in this case, by reducing its ability to fight viruses, and shrink tumors.

The particular component of green tea that is most studied, and considered to be most protective against radiation, is the polyphenol catechin known as EGCG (epigallocatechin-3 gallate). In animal studies, EGCG protected mice from whole-body radiation, both blocking lipid oxidation, and prolonging their life span. This component of green tea especially protected cells in the intestine, and hair follicles, from the damaging effects of radiation.

Yet, one study concluded, "The results indicate that Green Tea and Green Tea Polyphenols may have a major radioprotective effect. Each one of the catechins was a much less effective radioprotector, suggesting that total extract or a mixture of GTPs may be more effective than individual catechins". (7)

This, again, confirms that using the whole plant, whether as brewed tea, or a non-standardized, whole-tea supplement, is the best approach to getting full value from green tea.

Shiitake Mushrooms

When looking to protect against radiation, shiitake mushrooms (Lentinula edodes) are another powerful, immune-enhancing food to add to the diet. Various mushrooms have been used to clean up contaminated radiation sites, an example of how well they absorb radiation. Around the Chernobyl site, the mushrooms that naturally grow there are considered toxic and inedible, and the wild pigs that do eat the mushrooms in turn have their flesh contaminated with radiation. Therefore, we should know where edible mushrooms are grown, before we purchase them (and, again, ideally they should be organic).

Macrophages are specialized cells that are an important component of our immune system. Their job is to identify and destroy other cells, which are potentially cancerous. These macrophage cells need to be activated in order to do their job, and shiitake mushrooms have been proven to activate these protective cells.

As well, shiitake mushrooms are naturally high in polysaccharides, another important immuno-supportive agent. Shiitake polysaccharides have been studied on laboratory animals, under a wide variety of circumstances, including exercise-induced stress, exposure to inflammation-producing toxins, radiation exposure, and immunodeficiency. In all cases, the polysaccharides in shiitake mushrooms have shown to help the immune system cope with these assaults. (8)

Soybeans

While many people are currently critical of all soy products (an issue I addressed in Health Secrets Volume One), soy does in fact contain many substances that support good health, some of which have radioprotective effects. However, soy foods in excess can block iodine uptake, and inhibit thyroid function. This can be a problem if you are not already consuming foods, or supplements, containing iodine. If you are consuming some iodine, then soy foods can be part of a healthy diet—if you are not allergic to them. The healthiest forms are the fermented products, miso, tamari, and tempeh, followed by tofu and soymilk (both of which are very cooling, and should be used in moderation).

Genistein, a component of soy known as an isoflavone, is known to protect mice from ionizing radiation damage. Genistein protects against radiation-induced lipid peroxidation, which causes damage by disrupting cell membranes and structures. As well, genistein stimulates production of red and white blood cells, following whole-body radiation exposure. (9)

Because some rat studies, which used genistein in isolation, have shown mixed results, it is best to get it in the form of soy foods, rather than in supplemental form (where it exists as an isolated component). While soy foods are the highest sources of genistein (especially soy flour, water-extracted soy protein concentrate, miso, dry roasted soybeans, and tempeh), other plant foods also contain some. These include alfalfa and clover sprouts, barley, broccoli, cauliflower, garbanzo beans, and sunflower seeds.

Sunflower Seeds

Like apples, raw sunflower seeds are high in the fiber pectin, which binds and removes radioactive particles from the body. Pectin is especially good at removing radioactive cesium-137, which collects in the endocrine glands, pancreas, thymus, and heart.

Sunflowers are so good at pulling radiation they have been used to clean contaminated soil. Sunflowers were planted all around the Chernobyl nuclear accident site for this purpose. Within six months of the Fukushima catastrophe, millions of sunflowers were planted in radioactive areas of Japan, in order to soak up radiation from the ground (and to visually make things look brighter, and more promising).

If you happen to have a garden on the West Coast exposed to the radioactive rain that fell during the first few weeks of the Fukushima accident, you may wish to revitalize your garden soil this way. Of course, you must discard the first crop of sunflowers, as they will not be fit to eat. One source maintained that sunflowers remove 95% of the radiation in soil within 20 days—whereas, it would normally take about 30 years until radiation levels reduced to a safe level.

Water

Currently, the best form of filtration for water is believed to be reverse osmosis. It will remove the majority of radioactive particles, as well removing heavy metals, microbial contaminants, and pesticides. RO water-filtration systems are commonly found in health food stores, and grocery stores, where customers fill their own bottles. Such units are also available in compact form, for home use, at reasonable prices. Since radiation is carried in steam coming off damaged nuclear reactors, we can assume that distillation may not be effective for these purposes.

A reverse osmosis water-filter forces the water through a membrane with small pores, with pressures ranging from 100 to 150 psi. Any molecules larger than the pore openings are removed from the water (a process that unfortunately wastes a significant portion of the water).

According to the U.S. EPA, reverse osmosis is the best available technology for removing uranium, radium, gross alpha, and beta particles, and photon emitters. They maintain it can remove up to 99% of these radionuclides.

Endnotes

1. Beneficial Biological Effects of Miso with Reference to Radiation Injury, Cancer and Hypertension." Hiromitsu Watanabe; J Toxicol Pathol. Jun 2013; 26(2): 91–103

2. Singh SP, et al. "Radioprotection of mice following garlic pre-treatment." Br J Cancer Suppl. 1996 Jul; 27:S102-4

3. "Radioprotective activity of betalains from red beets in mice exposed to gamma irradiation."; Eur J Pharmacol. 2009 Aug 1;615 (1-3):223-7

4. "Evaluation of the Radioprotective Action of Rutin in Mice Exposes to Gamma-Radiation."; Shrikant L. Patil. et al. / International Journal of Biological & Pharmaceutical Research. 2012; 3(1): 12-18

5. "Dietary flaxseed prevents radiation-induced oxidative lung damage, inflammation and fibrosis in a mouse model of thoracic radiation injury." Cancer Biol Ther. 2009 Jan;8(1):47-53; James C Lee, et al.

6. Venkatesh P, et al. "Ginger (Zingiber officinale Rosc.), a dietary supplement, protects mice against radiation-induced lethality: mechanism of action." Cancer Biother Radiopharm. 2004 Aug; 19 (4):422-35

7. Lee HJ, et al. "Modification of gamma-radiation response in mice by green tea polyphenols. "Phytother Res. 2008 Oct; 22 (10):1380-3

8. Kojima H, et al. "Structural analysis of glycogen-like polysaccharides having macrophage-activating activity in extracts of Lentinula edodes mycelia." J Nat Med. 2010 Jan; 64(1):16-23

9. Landauer MR, et al. "Genistein treatment protects mice from ionizing radiation injury." J Appl Toxicol. 2003 Nov-Dec; 23(6):379-85

RADIOPROTECTIVE SUPPLEMENTS

In this chapter, you will discover there are many supplements with a solid scientific basis, proving they can protect us from radiation damage. Most of the vitamins and minerals discussed should be used on a semi-regular basis (generally 5 days a week), since they are almost all required for general health needs in the body. However, we should take a different approach to the herbs, and superfoods (algae and grasses).

One approach is to choose which of these compounds to use based on other benefits they have, over and above fighting radiation damage. Thus, if you have memory problems you may pick gingko to use, and if you have asthma you might choose quercetin.

The other approach is to cycle the agents in question. So, for example, one month I might use burdock, and the next month I switch to ginseng. Then, the following month, I choose resveratrol. After which, I can rotate back to burdock, or move through the other options, perhaps observing their effects on my body. Eventually I can settle on those that offer me the widest benefits.

In either case, it is usually advisable to take a break from any given herb, since our bodies do have a tendency to habituate to the effects of herbs, if we use them for too long. Taking a break for a few weeks, or a month, or in this case, substituting with another herb that serves the similar function of protecting us against radiation, allows each herb to work at full effectiveness when we return to it.

As well, we should all probably be taking at least one of the green superfoods—as most of us do not eat enough vegetables to fully alkalize our bodies—and the cleansing ability of high-chlorophyll algae and grasses are unsurpassed. The superfoods do not need to be rotated, since they function more like foods than herbs. Though again, it may serve you to try different ones, until you find one, or two, that are most agreeable to your body.

CHLOROPHYLL

Chlorophyll is the pigment that gives plants their green color. It has a core of magnesium, and has a similar structure to hemoglobin, thus helping the body to build red blood cells. Its propensity for alkalizing, and detoxifying, the body, have lead it to be a mainstay in the health food industry, ultimately resulting in the prevalence of "green" drink mixes.

While chlorophyll alone, as a liquid supplement, has its value, more nutritional value is to be found when whole green plants are used. The most common sources of chlorophyll-rich foods used alone, or in green drinks, are the grasses and algae.

Especially helpful for removing radiation from the body are the cereal grasses—most commonly, barley and wheat grass. The juice concentrate of such grasses are more palatable than the ground grasses, as the gritty, insoluble fiber component is removed from the juices. Unlike using just liquid chlorophyll alone, the grasses are very high in minerals, and so are much more alkalizing. As well, they also contain enzymes, which work to clean the blood, and improve nutrient absorption.

A company that specializes in wheatgrass production once tested wheat grass against barley grass, to see which had more value. They concluded that, if they were grown in the same soil, there was no appreciable difference between the two—so for our purposes they may be used interchangeably.

It should be noted that indoor grown wheatgrass has far fewer minerals than outdoor grown. This is because the shoots of outdoor plants can reach deep into the soil, bringing up minerals into the body of the plant. Indoor grown grasses are also prone to picking up mold, which is very counterproductive to good health.

The other chlorophyll-rich superfoods particularly good for treating radiation contamination are algae—especially spirulina and chlorella. Both these algae were used by the Institute of Radiation Medicine in Russia, after Chernobyl, in order to enhance immunity, and balance blood chemistry, in victims of that crisis. Earthrise, an American spirulina company, provided spirulina to children contaminated during the Chernobyl crisis, to very positive effect. (1)

It is important to realize, when we use more than one variety of algae, or grass juice, it is best not to combine them at therapeutic dose levels. Thus, if you were using both barley grass (3-6 gr average daily dose), and wheat grass (3-6 gr average daily dose), you would take only half a recommended dose of each, and not a full serving. The same principle holds for stacking spirulina (3-6 gr), and chlorella (3-6 gr): your total intake of the combined algae would be 3 to 6 gr.

On the other hand, it would be all right to combine a full dose of algae with a full dose of a cereal grass, since they have different properties. Even so, the higher dosage of combinations should be worked up to gradually, since too much, too soon, can cause side effects (most commonly nausea, and skin breakouts), due to rapid detoxification.

Because algae grow in water, and grasses grow in earth, they have different properties, from the perspective of Chinese medicine. As a very general rule of thumb, algae best serves those with a diet high in animal protein, and the grasses work better for those with vegetarian, or vegan, diets. Algae are also better suited to the warmer seasons, and grasses to the colder, damp seasons.

MELATONIN

As mentioned in the chapter on melatonin, aside from regulating sleeping patterns, it also serves some antioxidant functions. In this case, it protects the body from the effects of radiation damage on DNA. Melatonin also protects dividing cells, and circulating blood cells, from chromosomal injury by radiation. (2) A daily dose of melatonin is from one to three mg, based on age (seniors require about 3 mg), and should be taken sublingually, just before bed.

QUERCETIN

Commonly used as a natural anti-histamine (especially for allergies and asthma), quercetin is a flavonoid, found in fruits, vegetables, and grains—one with powerful anti-inflammatory benefits. It will also protect lipids and proteins from dangerous doses of gamma radiation, mostly through its antioxidant properties.

Quercetin provides protection from chromosomal damage caused by radiation, and protects mitochondrial DNA from radiation-induced oxidant damage. As well, quercetin mitigates changes in human white blood cells, following radiation exposure. (3) Quercetin is commonly taken at a dose of 500 mg, one to three times daily, and is considered by some experts to be more effective when combined with bromelain.

RESVERATROL

Resveratrol, a well-researched antioxidant, and longevity agent, is found in fruits and vegetables, and particularly in red wine—with higher levels being found in organic wine. It is both radioprotective, and has antitumor activity. In mice studies, resveratrol protected mouse chromosomes from radiation-induced damage, and prevented radiation toxicity to the liver and small intestines—two areas very sensitive to damage from radiation. (4)

Resveratrol, in its active form, is known as "trans-resveratrol", and this the benchmark to look for on labels. Doses range from 50 to

250 mg of encapsulated trans-resveratrol, one to three times daily. However, liquid resveratrol, taken sublingually (under the tongue), will increase absorption by up to 50 times more than taking a pill. One excellent resveratrol product (that also includes turmeric extract) is Liposomal Curcumin/Resveratrol (from NutriStart Vitamin Company, in Canada). As this product is both liposomal, and sublingual, it is likely the best-absorbed resveratrol on the market.

RADIOPROTECTIVE HERBS

Astragalus

Astragalus has potent immuno-modulating, anti-allergenic, anti-microbial, antiviral, and adaptogenic properties. In Chinese Medicine, astragalus is used to strengthen the immune system, and prevent and treat common colds, and upper respiratory infections. As well, doctors of Chinese medicine use astragalus to reduce adverse effects of therapeutic radiation, and chemotherapy, in cancer patients.

There are certain drugs used to treat workers in the nuclear industry exposed to dangerously high amounts of radiation. These drugs, Neupogen and Neulasta, are blood-derived medications that increase the manufacture of white blood cells, encouraging the body to fight off infection.

The herb astragalus also has this ability to increase white blood cells, as well as being a superior immune supporter. Astragalus is extremely safe, even for children, and works best when taken as a tonic over long periods. This makes it an exception to the idea, mentioned previously, that herbs should be rotated, and not taken consistently over long periods of time.

In a lab study, astragalus extract "increased the survival rate of mice and made the damaged organ injured by irradiation recovered to normal appearance with the mechanism of enhancing immune function and blood-producing function". (5)

Recommended dose of astragalus:

Standardized extract: 250–500 mg, 3 times per day.

Decoction (strong boiled tea): 3–6 g of dried root per 12 oz water, 3 times per day.

Tincture (1:5) in 30% ethanol: 20–60 drops, 3 times per day.

Burdock Root

Burdock root, used as a food in parts of Asia but treated as a herb in the West, is considered a blood cleanser, and a "cooling" liver tonic. It is used traditionally to treat skin conditions such as dermatitis, eczema, and psoriasis. Burdock Root also helps remove radioactive isotopes from the body, and can prevent and reverse DNA damage done by radiation exposure.

Burdock can be used in cooking, or juiced (fresh burdock), or consumed as a tea (fresh or dried). It can be taken as a tincture, or in capsule form (follow dosage instructions on label). A therapeutic dose is 1 to 4 ounces of fresh burdock root, or a teaspoon of dried root. Ideally, raw burdock is the best choice since enzymes are present (offering additional benefits), but tea, tincture, and capsules will still be effective for our purposes.

Traditional blood-cleansing formulas will help relieve the toxic load on the body, allowing it to cope better with the extra burden of radiation. Based on the most powerful herbal blood cleansers (red clover and burdock), formulas such as the Hoxey Formula (which includes potassium iodide), and Essiac, have been used as alternative cancer treatments for many decades. The best such formula available is "Flor-Essence" (which also includes kelp), a modern variation on the Essiac formula, produced by Flora Health Company.

As a bonus, my research on burdock found a study indicating that an "aqueous (water) extract of Arctium lappa (burdock) roots enhances sexual behavior in male rats…These results thus support the traditional use of Arctium lappa L. root extract for treating impotence and sterility". (6)

Echinacea

Like many, I have used echinacea tincture as a cold and flu remedy for years. I find it highly effective for either preventing a cold, or shortening the duration of it, as well as for alleviating symptoms. I have found people who think echinacea does not work usually do not use enough of it: scientific material on effectiveness of echinacea is based on taking at least 30 drops, six times per day.

Echinacea does two things when fighting infection of any kind: it attacks and destroys invading bacteria, and enhances the functions of the immune system. This offers a two-pronged approach to dealing with bacterial or viral infections. Now, it turns out, echinacea has value when dealing with radiation exposure, as well.

A small-scale study focused on a group whose work included regular exposure to ionizing radiation. Ten male subjects were given two tablets of echinacea purpurea (275 mg each) twice a day, for two weeks. Throughout the study, the 10 subjects used no other drugs, or vitamin supplements.

The echinacea purpurea (a species of echinacea that is a better immune stimulant than the angustifolia species) was standardized to 8.3% total phenolic content (calculated in terms of chlorogenic acid units).

This study concluded the echinacea purpurea supplement "significantly reduces the incidence of radiation-induced chromosomal aberrations and micronuclei (a characteristic of cells that exhibit DNA damage) in human lymphocytes of radiation workers. Its powerful radioprotective capacities are achieved through free radical scavenging performed by polyphenols, which stimulate apoptosis (programmed cell death designed to rid the body of unhealthy cells) and enhance monocyte-macrophage (type of white blood cell) activity". [7]

Be aware, when using echinacea in a tablet or capsule form, only the root, or concentrated extract of the flower, works. The flower itself only works when freshly made into a tincture—which can then be spray dried onto some medium, and encapsulated—and will not be effective when taken as a tea, or dried and put into pill form.

Ginkgo

Ginkgo biloba is mostly used as a mental aid to memory and cognition, effective because it enhances circulation and blood flow to the extremities (in this case to the brain), where it delivers more oxygen. This ability to enhance circulation has proven to be effective for treating impotency as well.

Ginkgo also functions as an antioxidant, which may be why it reduces DNA damage to people, and animals, exposed to radiation. In fact, ginkgo was used effectively to treat workers at the Chernobyl nuclear plant, even well after their initial exposure. More recent studies have proven ginkgo extracts protect animals' organs from direct radiation-induced damage, and humans from cell damage, following radioactive iodine treatment. (8)

Much of the ginkgo on the market has proven to be ineffective, so when purchasing a product be sure to look into the quality of it. (Two proven brands are Nature's Way Ginkgold, and A. Vogel gingko tablets, or tincture.)

Almost all clinical trials of ginkgo have used an extract of ginkgo, standardized to 24% flavone glycosides, and 6% terpene lactones. The most common dose used in these studies (including for people with dementia) is 40 mg of that standardized extract, three times daily. For improving cognitive function in healthy people, studies have used from 120 to 600 mg of the extract, daily.

Ginseng

Among the most useful herbs for coping with radiation in the body are members of the ginseng family: panax ginseng, grown in China and Korea; North American ginseng (panax quinque folium); and Siberian ginseng (eleutherococcus senticosus), which is not a true member of the ginseng family.

The ginseng-related herbs are known as adaptogens. Adaptogens are defined as substances that help an organism deal with stress: emotional, mental, physical, and/or toxic.

Early panax ginseng studies allowed science to believe the Asians may be onto something with their ginseng fascination, and led to the discovery of many more adaptogenic substances. In fact, almost every country (or culture) has some herb that is considered an adaptogen, and which has been used traditionally for longevity, and vitality.

Asian ginsengs have been used to improve the immunity of cancer patients, as well as reversing low white blood cell count, caused by chemotherapy, and radiation therapy. Siberian ginseng also has reversed suppression of white blood cells, and bone marrow, in cancer patients, as well as showing anti-tumor effects in vitro. (9)

Now, these three ginsengs have slightly different secondary attributes that one should be aware of before using. In Chinese medicine, "red" panax ginseng is considered "heating", and thus could aggravate high blood pressure, or hot flashes. On the other hand, North American ginseng is "cooling" and would be helpful in treating such heated conditions.

Panax ginseng, that is not processed to be "red", is only "warming" in nature, and Siberian ginseng is even less warming, and almost "neutral" in nature. Unless one knows (generally via a Chinese medicine practitioner) if one has a heated, or cooled (or "deficient") nature, one is advised to stick with non-red panax ginseng, or Siberian ginseng, which are both safe for long-term use.

Because panax ginseng is an expensive root, there is a risk of disreputable manufacturers selling adulterated products. Therefore, always buy from a company you can trust (or ensure that it is organic). This is not an issue with Siberian ginseng, since it is far less expensive than true ginseng.

According to the Complete German Commission E Monographs (international herbal standards), dried root powder of ginseng is used at a dosage of 1 to 2 gr daily, for up to 3 months. In clinical trials, the dosage of crude root has ranged from 0.5 to 3 g/day, and the dose of extracts has generally ranged from 100 to 400 mg daily.

Siberian ginseng extracts should be standardized to contain at least 0.8% eleutherosides (the active component). The dosage of such a product is from 100 to 200 mg, three times a day.

Holy Basil

The Ayurvedic (East Indian) herb holy basil (Tulsi), is commonly recommended for adrenal support, mood enhancement, and stress reduction. Recent research has indicated it is also very effective at protecting against radiation damage. Water-based, holy basil extracts, enhance survival of mice exposed to whole-body gamma radiation—much more effectively than alcoholic extracts (tincture). This suggests the radioprotective properties of holy basil are easily available when it is simply brewed as a tea. (10) Holy basil is also available in capsule form, and recommended dose for neurological, and adaptogenic, effects is 500 mg of the leaf extract, taken twice daily.

Milk Thistle

Milk thistle is well known for its ability to detoxify and protect the liver, and the liver handles the majority of the body's burden of toxins. Since milk thistle also raises glutathione levels in the liver, it is no surprise that it would facilitate the body coping with undue amounts of radiation.

Silymarin (the active component of milk thistle) has been shown to protect liver tissue from radiation damage, reduce DNA damage, and extend survival times in animals exposed to high levels of radiation. (11)

Most milk thistle products are standardized to 80% silymarin, and a therapeutic dose begins at 150 mg of silymarin, three times daily—though for severe liver damage, dosages have ranged up to 800 mg of silymarin daily (in divided doses). As with all herbs, it is best to take milk thistle daily for a month or so, and then take some time off (2–4 weeks), before returning to it.

For those with liver damage (such as cirrhosis or hepatitis), I find the best approach is to use a milk thistle product for one month, then switch over to a different form of liver-support for the following month. One can then cycle back to the milk thistle, and continue alternating. Alternative liver support products include those which are Ayurvedic (like Himalaya LiverCare), or those comprised of medicinal mushrooms. Another clinically proven liver supportive, Liverite Liver Aid, is an extract derived from cow liver.

Medicinal Mushrooms

Medicinal mushrooms can be of great value here, but we must ensure they are grown organically. Medicinal mushrooms come in a variety of combinations, and in various extraction forms (alcohol or steam extracted, micronized, standardized, etc.), so for dosage, follow label recommendations.

These therapeutic mushrooms contain a variety of substances, including glucans, beta-glucans, and heteropolysaccharides—all of which are powerful immune-modulators, and anti-tumor agents. These compounds are proven to improve the recovery of bone marrow, and limit blood changes, induced by radiation.

Reishi mushroom (ganoderma lucidum) can prolong the lives of cancer patients undergoing radiation therapy, indicating clear value here. (12) Reishi is also a wonderful tonic that benefits the lungs, liver, kidneys, and adrenal glands.

Another helpful medicinal mushroom is cordyceps (ophiocordyceps sinensis), which increases glutathione in the liver, and supports the adrenal glands, and "kidney essence" (an indicator of longevity, in Chinese medicine). Other mushrooms of particular value here include maitake (grifola frondosa), turkey tail (trametes versicolor), and zhu ling (polyporus umbellatus).

A few mushrooms are high in the substance melanin. (Melanin is a broad term for a group of natural pigments, found in most organisms, which gives color and tan to our skin.)

In a 2012 study, scientists fed mice a mushroom used in East Asian cuisine, called Judas' ear, or jelly ear (auricularia auricular), an hour before giving them a powerful dose of radioactive cesium137. All the control mice died in 13 days, but 90% of the mice fed this mushroom survived. Mice fed white mushrooms died almost as fast as the controls, but those fed white mushrooms supplemented with synthetic melanin also survived.

The study concluded that, "...local GI protection (shielding) with melanin-containing mushrooms translated into systemic protection, and this observation establishes a new concept in the approach for protecting against radiation syndrome. We anticipate that black edible mushrooms could be developed into low-cost oral radioprotectors for patients and affected populations exposed to ionizing radiation". (13)

Now, while this mushroom is not common in the West, an alternative is the chaga mushroom (inonotus obliquus), which happens to contain 25% melanin by dry weight. Chaga is commonly available in health food stores, and online, in a variety of user-friendly forms (capsules, tea, tincture), and has many other valuable medicinal properties. These include being an antioxidant, regulating insulin, enhancing immune function, protecting the liver, reducing inflammation, and preventing cancer and tumor formation.

Rosemary

Rosemary contains compounds (carnosic acid and carnosol) which work against the mutagenic effects of radiation. In one study, where mice were exposed to radiation, the results were remarkable: the animals given rosemary extract regained normal parameters of health after 30 days, whereas the mice in the control group never attained normal values.

To quote from that study, "In control animals, there was an

elevation in lipid peroxidation (LPx) and a decrease in glutathione (GSH) in blood and liver; whereas in the experimental group, decline in LPx accompanied by an increase in GSH concentration was observed". (14) Rosemary can be used liberally in cooking, and/or taken as a tea, or tincture.

Turmeric

Turmeric (whether used as a food or a supplement) has a solid traditional and scientific base of evidence showing it to be an anti-oxidant, anti-inflammatory, anti-depressant, and anti-cancer agent. As well, more recent studies have proven it also works to prevent diabetes, and Alzheimer's disease.

The most researched compound found in turmeric, curcumin, has potent radioprotective effects as a result of its powerful antioxidant functions, and its ability to modify gene expression. Curcumin can even up-regulate genes responsible for destroying cancer cells, helping to shrink tumors.

Curcumin studies show it reduces DNA damage and tumor formation in rats, and increases survival times in animals exposed to high levels of radiation. Also, in cultured human white blood cells, curcumin reduces DNA damage and lipid peroxidation, both symptoms of radiation damage. (15)

Turmeric can be used in cooking, but for therapeutic effects, you will need to ingest about a tablespoon of powder over the course of a day. Since its nutritive elements are mostly fat-soluble, turmeric ideally should be used with meals containing fat. Below is the recipe for "Golden Paste" a popular way of using turmeric powder in a fat-based medium.

In a saucepan add ½ cup of organic turmeric powder to 1 cup of water (filtered or spring), and gently stir and heat (for 5 – 10 minutes) until you get a thick paste. You can add more water or turmeric to get the right consistency. Next add ½ to 1 teaspoon of freshly ground black pepper, and ¼ cup of either extra virgin olive oil or coconut oil (either refined or virgin will work). Continue stirring until all ingredients are well mixed, then set aside to cool. Keep in a glass jar in the fridge for up to 2 weeks.

A serving is from ¼ to ½ teaspoon, to be taken three or more times daily, if trying to control inflammation, or treat a health condition. Otherwise, one may take as much as is palatable, in any manner chosen.

Turmeric paste can be taken directly off the spoon into the mouth, or mixed with honey, to improve the taste. Alternatively, it can be mixed into hot water, or added to herbal teas, hot milk, or almond milk, with a bit of natural sweetener. It can also be mixed into grains, pasta, soup, or savory dishes, either during the cooking process, or at the table. Finally, it can be blended into smoothies, or protein shakes.

Most turmeric supplements of value are in a base of oil, but should still be taken with meals containing fat. However, there is now a well-researched, water-soluble version of turmeric extract, called "Theracurmin", which can be used without fat being present.

While there are many scientific studies on the effectiveness of curcumin, some studies have indicated that long-term use can increase free radical damage. This may occur because curcumin is one isolated fraction of the plant, and is missing its naturally occurring co-factors. For that reason, when purchasing turmeric extracts in supplemental form, you should look for products that concentrate the full range of "curcuminoids".

These products are usually standardized to 95% curcuminoids, and though the amount of curcumin may seem low, they are still highly effective products, and have been proven so in clinical studies. Dosage levels of turmeric products standardized to 95% curcuminoids (including Theracurmin), is from 500 to 750 mg, once or twice daily.

Other Herbs

Licorice extract prevents DNA damage, and protects lipids from radiation-induced peroxidation. (16) It is easy to consume as a tasty tea, or as licorice extract candies, available in health food stores. (However, be aware most licorice candies have very little, if any, actual licorice in them, so read the label.). Licorice can also be taken in capsule, or tincture, form, but should not be used without professional advice if you have high blood pressure.

A study published in the Journal of Clinical Biochemistry and Nutrition (2007), collected the best-researched radioprotective plants and herbal extracts, based on both in vitro and in vivo studies. They found the following herbs (excluding those we have already discussed) to "protect against radiation-induced lethality, lipid peroxidation and DNA damage".

Gotu kola (Centella asiatica); sea buckthorn (Hippophae rhamnoides); amla or Indian gooseberry (Emblica officinalis); Indian long pepper (Piper longum); field mint or wild mint (Mentha arvensis); peppermint (Mentha piperita). (17)

RADIOPROTECTIVE MINERALS

As well as eating a mineral-rich diet, it is also important to keep our supplemental mineral intake high, in order to support alkalinity. Here we will look at the most important minerals to consider supplementing with, when dealing with radiation issues.

Boron

The mineral boron is used by the nuclear industry to wash down leaking power plants, in order to trap radiation in the cooling water (which is then dumped into the ocean). It is used in nuclear power plants both to reduce pipe corrosion, and because it absorbs radiation very effectively.

Boron as a supplement is useful for treating arthritis, and osteoporosis, as well as for hormonal regulation in both genders. It is found in high amounts in organic apples, which, along with the pectin and calcium d-glucarate present, make this the superior fruit for protecting against radiation. The therapeutic dose of boron is 3 mg daily. (For an overview of the many benefits of boron, including anticancer properties, search Pubmed for the article titled "Nothing Boring About Boron".)

Calcium

Calcium protects against the absorption of radioactive strontium and uranium into the bones. If you are consuming dairy products on a regular basis, do not take more than 200 to 300 mg of elemental calcium daily. As I indicated in the previous volume of Health Secrets, too much calcium can be dangerous. If you do not regularly consume dairy products, you can take from 300 to 600 mg of elemental calcium (up to 5 days a week).

Iron

Iron inhibits absorption of plutonium, but dose should be based on age, and gender. Generally iron is only found in multivitamins meant for menstruating women, but not in those designed for men, or women past menstruation. This is because excess iron has been linked to heart disease, in those who eat red meat frequently. The best idea is to get a blood test to see if you need iron supplementation, or not.

Magnesium

Magnesium slows the influx of calcium ions, which in turn reduces the conversion of iodide to iodine. This is important during a radioactive emergency, when the body needs iodide (rather than iodine) in order to protect the thyroid from taking up radioactive iodine.

Average dose is from 400 to 600 mg elemental, daily, in divided doses. Magnesium is also a nutrient required by the body to deal with high levels of stress, which clearly would be an issue during a radioactive emergency.

Selenium

Selenium is required for the production of glutathione, and works synergistically with vitamin E as an antioxidant. Selenium also binds to mercury (rendering it less damaging, and reducing our total load of toxins), and is a powerful anti-viral agent. Personally, I do not recommend the use of selenomethionine, though it is currently a popular form. I prefer the selenium supplements derived from nutritional yeast, since they have proven to be safe, and effective, over a long period of time. The recommended daily dose of selenium is 100–200 mcg daily.

Strontium

The mineral strontium has an affinity for bones, and is taken up by the bones in a manner similar to how calcium is absorbed. It is therefore used to treat osteoporosis, but will also protect the body from taking up excess radioactive strontium-90: a specific byproduct of nuclear waste. Strontium-90 has a tendency to accumulate in milk, both in animals and humans, and, to a lesser degree, also builds up in meat, fish, and eggs. As a supplement, strontium is usually available in a dose of about 350 mg, which is taken once or twice per day (away from calcium, or dairy products).

Zinc and Manganese

Zinc and manganese are both important for sustaining whole-body resistance to ionizing radiation, in part because they are required for the production of glutathione, and superoxide dismutase (SOD). Zinc supplements have protected rats from free radical damage to their red blood cells, caused by radioactive iodine. And, zinc has also proven to protect bone marrow from radiation-induced damage, though, interestingly, did not protect tumor cells from such damage.

Mitochondria, our cellular energy factories, produce large amounts of free radicals as a byproduct of energy production, and they are especially susceptible to radiation damage. Animal studies have proven that zinc, along with manganese, provides mitochondria-specific radioprotection. (18)

The zinc requirements of men are twice that of women, but usually, if you are taking a gender-specific multivitamin product, there will be sufficient zinc to meet normal requirements. One obvious symptom of zinc deficiency is white spots on the fingernails, indicating that a higher level of supplementation will be required. On average, if one is not deficient, a woman should ingest from 10 to 15 mg of zinc daily, while men should average 20 to 30 mg.

Sulfur

Sulfur is a mineral, but not easily found in supplemental form. Therefore, we will look at a variety of ways to increase sulfur in our bodies, since sulfur prevents the uptake of radioactive sulfur-35.

MSM

One way to increase our intake of sulfur is to use MSM (methylsulfonyl methane), which is a natural sulfur compound available in pill or powder form (though the powder tastes quite bitter). MSM is a good anti-inflammatory, with additional benefits for tendons, ligaments, hair, skin, and preventing allergies. A dose of MSM runs from 2 to 6 gr daily, though more can be safely taken for serious pain issues.

DMSO

Dimethyl sulfoxide is a sulfur compound that has a wide range of therapeutic applications, with around 40 pharmacological properties. DMSO is mostly used topically (it enters the blood via the skin), usually for treating arthritis, and inflammation. The ingestion of DMSO orally should only be done with the guidance of a health professional, as it can be dangerous when taken in this manner.

A Japanese study showed that even low concentrations of DMSO had radioprotective effects by facilitating DNA double-strand break repair, providing protection against cellular radiation damage throughout the body. (19)

N-A-C

Another supplemental form of sulfur is N-Acetyl-Cysteine, which is one of the best glutathione boosters, also good for removing mucous from the lungs.

NAC reduces liver damage caused by radiation, and limits free radical and DNA damage, both before and after radiation exposure. NAC also stimulates the release of cytokines (chemical messengers), shown to protect bone marrow against radiation injury.

In one study, NAC was combined with a multivitamin mixture (including vitamins C and E), and the formula significantly increased 30-day survival of mice exposed to a potentially lethal dose of X-rays. The protective effect was the same whether the supplement was given before, or after, the exposure to radiation. (20)

Dosage for NAC is 500 mg, one to three times daily. Do not take more than 1,500 mg daily, without the advice of a health professional— NAC has a tendency to create free radicals, when taken in excess.

RADIOPROTECTIVE VITAMINS

Radiation does most of its damage via free-radical production in the body—contributing to premature aging, cancer (especially leukemia), heart disease, birth defects, and more. Radiation therapy (and I use the term "therapy" very loosely) has been shown to deplete the body of beta carotene, and vitamins C and E. However, research on patients undergoing radiation therapy has proven that providing them with vitamins C and E reduces cellular damage caused by radiation.

ACES

The most important antioxidants are collectively known as the ACES, and include vitamins A (referring to beta-carotene, also known as pro-vitamin A), C and E, along with the mineral selenium (which works in a synergistic manner with the other antioxidants).

Many of the antioxidant compounds previously discussed—found in foods and herbs—may be more powerful free radical scavengers than the ACES. However, these four antioxidants are also essential nutrients. This means they serve many functions in the body, over and above just being free radical scavengers.

A high intake of the ACES, along with other antioxidants, have proven to protect airline pilots from radiation-induced chromosomal damage: an occupational hazard for those who work consistently at high altitudes. (21)

Vitamin A and Beta-Carotene

Beta-carotene, the precursor of vitamin A, was first used clinically to treat radiation damage in children, following the Chernobyl nuclear accident. Supplementation with beta-carotene reduced the amount of radiation-induced oxidized lipids in these children. (22)

Beta-carotene is a more powerful antioxidant than vitamin A, but the latter is essential to maintaining our mucous membranes (which can be damaged by radiation). The body will convert some beta-carotene into vitamin A, but we can never be sure if it is enough. Since the only appreciable food source of vitamin A is liver (from fish or mammals), I would advise most people, who do not eat liver on a regular basis, to supplement with vitamin A.

The Albert Einstein College of Medicine, in 1984, reported that both vitamin A, and beta-carotene, counteracted total body gamma radiation. While dealing with radiation poisoning, these nutrients helped to reduce weight loss, and inhibit abnormal decreases in red and white blood cell formation. As well, they prevented adrenal enlargement, atrophy of the thymus gland and spleen, and ulceration of the gastrointestinal tract.

Controlled animal studies also showed vitamin A could reverse radiation-induced gene expression abnormalities that lead to cancer, and can even destroy cancerous cells. (23)

A maintenance dose of Vitamin A is 10,000 IU daily (5 days a week). For therapeutic purposes, 30,000 to 50,000 IU is the recommended dose for adults, for short-term usage (a few weeks). During emergencies, or crisis situations, intensive exposure to radiation may require even higher amounts (even up to 100,000 IU, briefly).

It should be noted when we take vitamin A together with beta-carotene, we free up the beta-carotene to only scavenge free radicals. Having fulfilled the body's requirement for vitamin A, none of the beta-carotene will need to be converted into vitamin A.

The recommended dose of beta-carotene is 25,000 IU once or twice daily. Beta-carotene as a supplement should always be derived from natural sources, and such products will include the whole family of carotenoids. (Two such brands are BetaCareAll and Betatene.) Synthetic beta-carotene (found in most multivitamins) is known to increase cancer risk, especially in smokers.

Vitamin C

Vitamin C inhibits radiation-induced death of human blood cells, and can counteract radiation-induced "long-lived radicals" that destabilize chromosomes, and induce cancerous mutations. This ability to counteract both general free radicals, as well as long-lived free radicals, is critical to preventing genetic damage from radiation. (24)

A minimum dose for vitamin C is 500–1000 mg, three times daily, either as ascorbic acid, or in the "buffered" form (e.g. calcium ascorbate). Any buffered vitamin C (or "mineral ascorbate") will stay in the blood longer than ascorbic acid. One may safely take much more vitamin C than that, if desired, though too much ascorbic acid will cause a laxative effect. And, if taking more than a few grams daily, avoid calcium ascorbate, as this form can add too much calcium to your daily intake (each gram provides 90 mg of calcium).

Vitamin E

Vitamin E (alpha tocopherol) helps to prevent damage to cell membranes caused by ionizing radiation. It works by preventing chain reactions triggered by radiation, which oxidize the polyunsaturated lipids in cell membranes—the same mechanism that makes fats go rancid. Radiation damage essentially causes the cell membranes to go rancid, leading to most of the damage to the rest of the cell, and to its DNA.

Like vitamin C, and beta-carotene, vitamin E stabilizes free radicals once they form, reducing the amount of damage radiation can do. In fact, animal studies show vitamin E significantly protects mice from dying, after exposure to lethal levels of gamma rays. And, not only did vitamin E help protect the animals from radiation damage, it also increased new blood cell formation which had been suppressed by the radiation. (25)

When supplementing with vitamin E, it is essential to get one derived from a natural source, and ideally, in a "mixed" form. Mixed vitamin E contains alpha tocopherol, along with appreciable amounts of beta, gamma, and delta tocopherols—the rest of the vitamin E "family". A maintenance dose is from 400 to 800 IU daily.

Vitamin B-12

This nutrient inhibits the uptake of radioactive cobalt because it is a form of cobalt (either in the cyanocobalamin or methylcobalamin forms). Thus, B-12 can occupy the receptor sites this type of radiation would attempt to attach to. Maintenance dose is between 100 mcg and 1 mg of B-12, daily, the amount being based on a number of factors, including age, health, and diet. Ideally one uses B-12 in the methylcobalamin form, which should be taken sublingually (under the tongue), or by injection (in the case of severe health problems).

PROBIOTICS

By now, most of us know the value of ingesting fermented foods, and/or probiotic supplements, in order to keep a healthy supply of friendly flora in our intestines. Ailments linked to an imbalance of good and bad bacteria in the gut, range from digestive and bowel-related disorders, to neurological conditions, including autism, anxiety, and depression.

A healthy profile of good bacteria is also essential to having a well-functioning immune system. Therefore, it makes sense probiotics could help us cope with the damaging effects of radiation exposure. And, as we will see, some studies clearly indicate specific probiotics can directly help the body cope with radiation.

A Bulgarian product called Biomilk (a modern form of traditional Bulgarian yogurt), is rich in the probiotic species known as Lactobacillus bulgaricus (currently the scientific name is Lactobacillus delbrueckii, subspecies bulgaricus). This bacteria is one of several used for the production of yogurt and Swiss cheese.

Bulgarian studies show the use of Biomilk reduces the degree of injury to bone marrow, has a radioprotective effect on stem cells, and reduces rates of mortality, in experimental animals given lethal doses of radiation. The researchers assumed that, "Most likely the radioprotective effect of Biomilk with Lactobacillus bulgaricus is due to its immuno-stimulating effect and the fact that it limits the lipid peroxidation, i.e. reduction of the free radicals". (26)

In humans, cancer patients who took Biomilk endured radiation, and chemotherapy, better than those who did not, and had better survival times. It is also claimed this product is so effective, it was used by astronauts from the international space program, Intercosmos (1978 -1988), to help protect them from radiation damage. (www.bio-milk.com)

Another probiotic found to protect against radiation damage was Lactobacillus rhamnosus. In research done at Washington University School of Medicine, scientists studied mice in order to determine if taking a probiotic might help cancer patients avoid intestinal injury—when receiving radiation therapy for abdominal cancers.

This study found that, in mice receiving radiation, L. rhamnosus (found mostly in dairy products, or probiotic supplements) protected the lining of the small intestine. However, in this case, researchers found that L. rhamnosus was effective only if given to mice before radiation exposure. If mice received the probiotic after damage to intestinal lining had occurred, the probiotic treatment could not repair the damage.

The head of this study concluded, "The bacteria we use is similar to what's found in yogurt or in commercially available probiotics. So theoretically, there shouldn't be risk associated with this preventive treatment strategy any more than there would be in a patient with abdominal cancer eating yogurt". (27)

Now, this final study I would not normally include, because the product used is both unusually strong, and unusually expensive. VSL#3 is a proprietary formulation of eight different probiotics (including L. bulgaricus), often used in combination with conventional therapies, to treat ulcerative colitis, and other bowel conditions. (www.vsl3.com)

A box of VSL#3 contains 30 packets, each pack contains 450 billion bacteria, and the product retails for about $190 CAD. So, this is not your everyday probiotic (though the feedback from those with chronic bowel conditions is very good).

I included this study because, unlike the previous one, it showed protective benefit even when not taken prior to radiation exposure. Though one could theorize, it is possible the last study used a dose too low to be of benefit after radiation exposure.

As with the previous study, the aim of this one was "to investigate the efficacy of a high-potency probiotic preparation on prevention of radiation-induced diarrhea in cancer patients". In this double-blind, placebo-controlled trial, 490 patients, who underwent postoperative radiation therapy after surgery for intestinal, rectal, or cervical cancer, were given either one packet of VSL#3, or placebo, beginning on the first day of radiation therapy.

The result was more placebo patients had radiation-induced diarrhea than VSL#3 patients (51.8% vs 31.6%), and more patients given placebo suffered grade 3 or 4 diarrhea (severe), compared with VSL#3 recipients (55.4% vs 1.4%).

In concluding that, "probiotic lactic acid-producing bacteria are an easy, safe, and feasible approach to protect cancer patients against the risk of radiation-induced diarrhea," there was no mention that L. bulgaricus was perhaps the most important bacteria in the formula.

All probiotics, including spore-based ones like bacillus coagulans (Lactospore)—as well as fermented foods—increase lactic acid levels in the intestines. This in turn feeds all good bacteria in your gut, encouraging them to colonize. The takeaway here is to consume many forms of fermented foods, and probiotics, on a regular basis. (28)

CLAY AND BAKING SODA

Bentonite clay (calcium bentonite being the preferred form), and French green clay (Montmorillonite), can attract and pull radiation from the body, when used internally, or externally. Clay works well because it has a negative ionic charge, and radioactive material has a positive ionic charge.

A Swedish study showed another kind of clay, called zeolite, could decontaminate live animals, and meat, affected by the Chernobyl meltdown. Most nuclear waste is currently mixed with zeolite clay, before being stored underground, because it helps prevent radioactivity from seeping into the ground after extended periods of time.

Recently, some commercial zeolite products were found to contain high amounts of lead, so be sure you buy a reputable product that has addressed this issue, if you wish to ingest it.

The usual approach, for internal use, is to mix a teaspoon of clay into water, let it settle, and drink the cloudy water, while leaving the sediment behind. One can work up to a teaspoon three times per day, for more therapeutic purposes. Ingesting clay should be done on an empty stomach (at least a half-hour before eating, or an hour after). Clays have also proved effective for removing heavy metals, purifying the intestinal tract, and alkalizing the body.

As well as being ingested, clay can also be used in a bath to remove radiation from the body. Simply add 1-2 cups of green clay, or bentonite, to a conventional-sized bath, and mix until dissolved. Ensure you remain in the hot bath for at least 20 minutes, and rinse off with cool water. You may add cold water during this process, but do not add more hot water once you have entered the bath.

Another bathing mixture, used for decontaminating radiation, is a combination of one cup of sea salt (or Himalayan salt) along with one cup of baking soda. Again, remain in the bath for at least 20 minutes, and rinse off with cool water. Baking soda alone can be used for this purpose, in which case one uses from one to 3 cups per bath (based on severity of exposure).

When taking a bath to remove radiation, it is important one leave the bath before draining the water out. Since radiation will follow the highest density object, as soon as your body weights more than the water remaining in the tub, the radiation will return to your body—rather than following the water down the drain.

Baking soda can also be used internally, and is recommended by the U.S. military for those exposed to radiation. Taken orally, baking soda can reduce damage uranium causes to the kidneys, and is a quick way to alkalize the body. Use ½ teaspoon of baking soda in purified water, on an empty stomach, three times daily.

If bathing in baking soda, clay, and/or salt can remove radiation from the skin, logic suggests this may also work on foodstuffs. In a situation where radiation is in the rain (as it was on the Pacific coast, following the Fukushima accident), it can contaminate produce still in the ground. It may make sense to soak fresh, wide-leafed vegetables, in a similar solution, if we suspect they have been exposed to radiation. Other fruits and vegetables exposed to radioactive rain should be peeled.

Borax (as used for washing clothes) is a form of boron, and in a pinch can be used in the bath (2-4 tbsp) to help remove radiation. It is also safe to wash vegetables in, and when used in the laundry will help to remove radiation from clothes exposed to radioactive rain.

During any crisis when radiation has become airborne, we should try to avoid exposure to rainfall. Heavy rain has measurably high levels of radiation in it, and if allowed to get into your eyes, or mouth, or to dry on the skin, it will absorb into the body. Also, remember that umbrellas and rain gear would then need to be washed in some of the above listed compounds, in order to remove radiation.

Endnotes

1. Qishen P, et al. "Radioprotective effect of extract from Spirulina platensis in mouse bone marrow cells studied by using the micronucleus test." Toxicol Lett. 1989 Aug; 48(2):165-9.

2. Koc M, et al. "The effect of melatonin on peripheral blood cells during total body irradiation in rats." Biol Pharm Bull. 2002 May; 25(5):656-7.

3. Devipriya N, et al. "Quercetin ameliorates gamma radiation-induced DNA damage and biochemical changes in human peripheral blood lymphocytes." Mutat Res. 2008 Jun 30; 654 (1):1-7.

4. Carsten RE, et al. "Resveratrol reduces radiation-induced chromosome aberration frequencies in mouse bone marrow cells." Radiat Res. 2008 Jun; 169(6):633-8.

5. Fitoterapia. 2011 Apr; 82(3):383-92.; "Protective effect of flavonoids from Astragalus complanatus on radiation induced damages in mice." Qi L, et al.

6. BMC Complement Altern Med. 2012 Feb 1; 12:8. "Effect of aqueous extract of Arctium lappa L. (burdock) roots on the sexual behavior of male rats." JianFeng C, et al.

7. Joksić G, et al. "Radioprotective Effects of Echinacea Purpurea." Arh Hig Rada Toksikol 2009; 60:165-172.

8. Emerit I, et al. "Clastogenic factors in the plasma of Chernobyl accident recovery workers: anticlastogenic effect of Ginkgo biloba extract." Radiat Res. 1995 Nov; 144(2):198-205.

9. Lee TK, et al. "Radioprotective potential of ginseng." Mutagenesis. 2005; 20:237–243.

10. Uma Devi, P., et al. "Radiation protection by the Ocimum flavonoids orientin and vicenin: Mechanisms of action." Radiation Research, 2000. 154(4): p. 455-460.

11. Ramadan LA, et al. "Radioprotective effect of silymarin against radiation induced hepatotoxicity." Pharmacol Res. 2002 Jun; 45(6):447-54.

12. Thulasi G, et al. "Polysaccharides isolated from Ganoderma lucidum occurring in Southern parts of India, protects radiation induced damages both in vitro and in vivo." Environmental Toxicology and Pharmacology 26 (2008) 80–85.

13. Cancer Biother Radiopharm. 2012 Nov; 27(9): 570–576. "Compton Scattering by Internal Shields Based on Melanin-Containing Mushrooms Provides Protection of Gastrointestinal Tract from Ionizing Radiation." Ekaterina Revskaya, et al.

14. Phytomedicine. 2007 Oct; 14(10):701-5; "Modulation of radiation-induced biochemical alterations in mice by rosemary (Rosemarinus officinalis) extract." Soyal D, et al.

15. Srinivasan M, et al. "Protective effect of curcumin on gamma-radiation induced DNA damage and lipid peroxidation in cultured human lymphocytes." Mutat Res. 2006 Dec 10; 611(1-2):96-103.

16. Shetty TK, et al. "Protection of DNA and microsomal membranes in vitro by Glycyrrhiza glabra L. against gamma irradiation." Phytother Res. 2002 Sep; 16(6):576-8.

17. "Radioprotective Potential of Plants and Herbs against the Effects of Ionizing Radiation." Ganesh C. Jagetia; J Clin Biochem Nutr. Mar 2007; 40(2): 74–8.

18. Floersheim GL, et al. "Differential radioprotection of bone marrow and tumour cells by zinc aspartate." Br J Radiol. 1988 Jun; 61(726):501-8.

19. J Radiat Res. 2010; 51(6):733-40; "An alternative mechanism for radioprotection by dimethyl sulfoxide; possible facilitation of DNA double-strand break repair." Kashino G1, et al.

20. Demirel C, et al. "Effect of N-acetylcysteine on radiation-induced genotoxicity and cytotoxicity in rat bone marrow." J Radiat Res (Tokyo). 2009 Jan; 50(1):43-50.

21. Yong LC, et al. "High dietary antioxidant intakes are associated with decreased chromosome translocation frequency in airline pilots." Am J Clin Nutr. 2009 Nov; 90(5):1402-10.

22. Ben-Amotz A, et al. "Effect of natural beta-carotene supplementation in children exposed to radiation from the Chernobyl accident." Radiat Environ Biophys. 1998 Oct;37(3):187-93.

23. J Nutr. 1998 Oct; 128(10):1661-4. "Vitamin A inhibits radiation-induced pneumonitis in rats."Redlich CA, et al.

24. Konopacka M, et al. "Inhibitory effect of ascorbic acid post-treatment on radiation-induced chromosomal damage in human lymphocytes in vitro." Teratog Carcinog Mutagen. 2002; 22(6):443-50.

25. Singh VK, et al. "Alpha-tocopherol succinate protects mice from gamma-radiation by induction of granulocyte-colony stimulating factor." Int J Radiat Biol. 2010 Jan; 86(1):12-21.

26. Medical Journal: Military Medicine 2007. "RAY-PROTECTIVE EFFECT OF THE PROBIOTIC BIOMILK." M. Georgieva. Department of preclinical and clinical pharmacology and biochemistry – Medical University Dr. Paraskev Stoyanov.

27. Ann N Y Acad Sci. 2009 May; 1165: 190–194. "Probiotic Therapy in Radiation-Induced Intestinal Injury and Repair." Matthew A. Ciorba and William F. Stenson.

28. World J Gastroenterol. 2007 Feb 14; 13(6): 912–915. "Use of probiotics for prevention of radiation-induced diarrhea." P Delia, G Sansotta, et al.

XENOESTROGENS

In the world of invisible agents assaulting our health, some of the most dangerous are chemicals that mimic our hormones. Hormone-disrupting chemicals are found everywhere in modern times, due to the prevalence of pesticides, preservatives, and plastics. Such chemicals are known as xenoestrogens, because they mimic the hormone estrogen. This mimicking of a natural hormone allows the chemicals easy access to the human (and animal) body.

ESTOGEN-MIMICKING CHEMICALS

We generally think of estrogen as a female hormone, but it is also present in, and necessary for, men as well (albeit in much lower amounts). Thus, men too have estrogen receptors.

Xenoestrogens block, or enhance, the effects of estrogen in the body, by binding to estrogen receptors. Excess estrogen (even the more natural form used in Estrogen Replacement Therapy), is linked to increased rates of cancer, as well as numerous other ailments.

Unlike natural estrogen produced by the body, or phyto-estrogenic compounds found in foods, xenoestrogens have a tendency to stay in the body and remain active for a much longer time. This gives them the opportunity to do enormous damage to us.

Estrogen, as it naturally occurs, is responsible, in women, for stimulating cell division in hormone sensitive tissues, including breast tissue, ovaries, and lining of the uterus. When mimicking xenoestrogens run amok in the body, they over-stimulate tissue growth in these hormone sensitive areas. This can lead to potential problems such as endometriosis, fibrocystic breast disease, ovarian cysts, polycystic ovarian syndrome, and breast cancer (as well as prostate cancer in men). Endometriosis and polycystic ovarian syndrome are also causes of infertility in women.

In areas where levels of compounds containing xenoestrogens (dioxins, bisphenol A, phthalates, organochlorine pesticides including PCB's, DDT, and lindane) are found to be high in the soil and water, we also find higher than normal breast cancer rates. (And those things which cause breast cancer also often cause prostate cancer.) Substances like these are known as endocrine disruptors, which means they interfere with the body's normal hormone signals. Thus, they can damage the immune system, and affect fertility, reproduction, and childhood development.

FERTILITY

Because they can upset the normal, delicate hormonal balance in the body, xenoestrogens can cause infertility. Environmental studies indicate that animals, fish, and amphibians, which live in, or near, water contaminated with xenoestrogens, often show reproductive malfunctions, infertility, or mutated sex organs. This is one reason why we are seeing declining sperm counts, and increasing rates of infertility, in humans who live in the industrialized countries.

Estrogen dominance, a situation where estrogen over-rides progesterone in the body, is known to impede fertility in women. This can naturally occur, but can also be caused by the extra load of xenoestrogens, leading to impairment of the luteal phase of fertility, and potentially causing miscarriages, and ectopic pregnancies. Xenoestrogens can also cross the placenta barrier, harming the fetus during development of the sex organs, and can migrate to breast milk, passing these chemicals on to the infant during nursing.

A hormone test can let a woman know if she has estrogen dominance, and if she does, one way to treat this condition is to use a naturally derived progesterone cream (about 20 mg a day).

Xenoestrogens also contribute to infertility, and low sperm count, in men, as well as to andropause symptoms (the male version of hormonal imbalance, akin to menopause in women). As a man's testosterone levels naturally decline with age, the extra estrogens he carries (whether naturally occurring, or from xenoestrogens), will proportionally rise in his blood—leading to emotional, mental, and physical symptoms. Researchers have also found a link between high xenoestrogens in the body, and low testosterone in men. (1)

So, once a man's testosterone starts to naturally decline, the presence of a high amount of xenoestrogens acts like a synthetic estrogen in his body. In men, low testosterone in combination with high estrogen, produces symptoms of increased body fat in the areas of the chest (gynecomastia), and abdomen (the most dangerous type of fat), along with loss of muscle mass. Other symptoms include depression, impotence, heart conditions, low sex drive, infertility, and prostate problems.

A man can also go to a doctor and get a hormone test to find out if his estrogen is too high, and/or his testosterone is too low. By working with a knowledgeable health professional, both men and women can re-establish a healthy hormone profile. This is accomplished by using natural substances that balance the necessary hormones, and by following some of the ideas presented further on, to block those hormones (or hormone-mimickers), that are in excess.

DIOXINS

One of the most common xenoestrogens found throughout the modern environment is dioxin. This byproduct of the industrial chlorine-bleaching process is used in creating diapers, menstrual pads, tampons, and white toilet paper (and is found in certain pesticides). When women use these bleached products regularly, the dioxins can be absorbed through their delicate mucous membranes (as with tampon use).

However, the vast majority of our exposure to dioxins is not from bleached products, but from food. Many commercially farmed dairy products, fish, meat, poultry, and shellfish, contain levels of dioxins well over the acceptable government standards. Of these, the World Health Organization (WHO) determined farmed fish to have the highest, most toxic levels of dioxins—far higher than dairy and meat.

Ailments linked to dioxin exposure include birth defects, diabetes, Hodgkin's disease, learning disabilities, non-Hodgkin's lymphoma, skin problems, soft-tissue cancers, and suppressed immune function. In fact, in 1997 the U.S. F.D.A. announced dioxin to be a cancer-causing agent to humans, confirmed, in that same year, by the World Health Organization. Even though these conclusions have since been repeatedly confirmed by research—leading to statements such as, "there is no safe level of dioxin exposure that is not linked to cancer"—dioxin is still commonly found in commercial foods, and continues to build up in the environment. (2)

Dioxins are also found in antibacterial ingredients such as triclosan (used in the new generation of antibacterial gels and soaps), and in PEG (polyethylene glycol) and related ethoxylated cleansers, such as sodium laureth sulfate (found in shampoos and other personal care products).

Unfortunately, dioxins, unlike another common xenoestrogen known as BPA (which the body can rid itself of relatively easily) stay in the body for long periods. It takes 11 years for dioxins to decay by half, and they are almost impossible to remove from the body with normal detoxification techniques, since they are very chemically stable, store in the fat cells, and do not break down easily.

ORGANOCHLORINES

Certain pesticides called organochlorines are organic compounds containing chlorine bonded to carbon, and are also considered xenoestrogens. These include DDT, dioxin, lindane (also used in lice medications), and atrazine. Organochlorines are also found in herbicides, detergents, spermicidal foam or lubricants, petrochemicals such as polychlorinated biphenyls (PCBs), PVC plastics, and some papers.

In the 1960s, experiments proved organochlorine pesticides caused breast cancer in rats, then, in the 1980s, another study concluded these pesticides "might be considered possible contributors to the high incidence of breast cancer among women".

More recently, scientists discovered women workers exposed to dioxin contamination had double the risk of breast cancer (chemical-plant workers in Hamburg, Germany). As well, higher levels of breast cancer were found in women living near organochlorine chemical plants in Minnesota, and Long Island. And, other studies have found elevated breast cancer rates among chemists, hairdressers, and users of hair dye (all of whom are also exposed to high levels of organochlorines).

Organochlorines are now found everywhere in the environment, including in animals and humans. Since organochlorines are stored in fat tissue, and poorly metabolized, they accumulate in the body. As a result, the amount of organochlorine in the bodies of animals becomes more and more concentrated, as they move up the food chain. Since humans are at the top of the food chain, we are storing dangerous amounts of organochlorines, in part, from the contaminated animals we eat.

PHTHALATES

Some of the worst xenoestrogen offenders are found in the plastics we use, in day-to-day living. Chief among these are the class of xenoestrogens known as phthalates, suspected of interfering with hormones, and with the reproductive development of baby boys (and which may be carcinogenic).

Cling-wrapped meats, cheeses, and other foods sold in delis and grocery stores, are wrapped in PVC (Polyvinyl chloride) plastic. During production, "plasticizers", known as adipates and phthalates, are added to polyvinyl chloride to soften the PVC into a flexible form. Traces of these chemicals can leak out of PVC when it comes in contact with foods—especially hot or fatty foods. These chemicals have been shown (in animal studies) to cause birth defects, and damage to the liver, kidneys, lungs, and reproductive systems.

A study on phthalates, done by Brigham and Women's Hospital, in Boston (published in the journal, Environmental Health Perspectives), analyzed urinary concentrations of phthalates in over 2,000 women, who were participating in the National Health and Nutrition Examination Survey. They found women with higher levels of phthalates in their urine were twice as likely to have diabetes, compared to women with the lowest levels of phthalates.

The women with higher than average urine levels of one form of phthalate (mono-3-carboxypropyl phthalate)—found in soaps, cosmetics and skin care products—had approximately a 60% increased risk of diabetes. While women who had moderately high levels of two other phthalates (mono-n-butyl phthalate, and di-2-ethylhexyl phthalate)—found in hair sprays, and gas-propelled personal care products—had approximately a 70% increased risk of diabetes.

CARS

Perhaps the worst exposure to phthalates occurs with that "new car smell", which is actually a gassing-off of phthalates from the initial heating up of a car full of plastic, glue, and synthetic carpets. These fumes also include the known carcinogens benzene and formaldehyde. Most of these gases dissipate in the first year, so for optimal health, one really does not want to purchase a brand new car, and, certainly not a new one every one or two years, as some do.

In a test of more than 200 vehicles, it was noted this off gassing of chemicals is notably lower in some cars, such as the Honda Civic, Toyota Prius, and Honda CR-Z.

Some of the newer cars that test well use no bromine-based flame-retardants in the interior components, use PVC-free interior fabrics and interior trim, and have low levels of heavy metals, and other metal allergens.

Those cars that scored poorly for toxins (including the Mitsubishi Outlander), contained bromine and antimony-based flame retardants in the seating, and center console, chromium-treated leather on several components, and lead in the seating materials.

According to the Ecology Center in Ann Arbor, Michigan, car manufacturers are beginning to reduce their use of chemicals, and some have eliminated flame-retardants and PVC plastics. They found that currently 17% of new vehicles have PVC-free interiors, and 60% are made without brominated flame-retardants. These chemicals, found on the armrests, dashboard, seats, and steering wheel, are easily absorbed into the body, and have been linked to numerous health problems, including allergies, impaired learning, and liver toxicity.

The real problem with these chemical and plastic compounds found in cars, is due to high temperatures increasing the concentration of VOCs (volatile organic compounds), and breaking other chemicals down into more toxic substances. "Automobiles function as chemical reactors, creating one of the most hazardous environments we spend time in," concluded the study from the Ecology Center.

You can find out how well, or poorly, a car rates for toxins, by going to healthystuff.org, and entering the name of the vehicle into their search engine.

AIR FRESHENERS

The regular use of synthetic air fresheners can cause health problems that include depression, earaches, headaches, and irregular heartbeat.

In 2007, the Natural Resources Defense Council released a report showing that 12 of 14 brands of household air fresheners contained phthalates. Phthalates are used in air fresheners to prolong the length of time these scented products maintain their fragrance. Unfortunately, some of the brands that tested positive for phthalates did not even include phthalates in their lists of ingredients, and some of these brands were even labeled as being "all-natural", and "unscented".

It should be pointed out, synthetic air fresheners which contain no phthalates, are still not safe to use in your car, or home. Most synthetic air fresheners still emit terpene, a VOC that reacts with naturally occurring ozone to create formaldehyde. (Formaldehyde is classified as a carcinogen by the International Agency for Research on Cancer.)

Since ozone is a form of oxygen that exists both indoors and outdoors, wherever synthetic air fresheners are used, there will be some formaldehyde formation (levels of ozone are especially high where photocopiers, and ozone-generating air-purifiers, are used).

In 2007, The American Journal of Respiratory and Critical Care Medicine published a study, based on collected data from 3,500 people, which showed regular use of air freshener sprays increase your risk of developing asthma by 30 to 50 percent.

Clearly, it is best to minimize our exposure to synthetic air fresheners, and other products designed to emit a prolonged artificial scent. After all, there are many natural air freshening options, including using essential oils in a diffuser.

AN ALTERNATIVE TO AIR FRESHENERS

One natural alternative to using air fresheners is to use bamboo charcoal pouches, which safely absorb odors, and chemicals. There are a few such products on the market, one of the better ones being airCOAL®, which is comprised of "100% Bamboo Charcoal in breathable Eco-fabric".

The big advantage of using charcoal pouches is they do not release potentially dangerous, odor-masking artificial fragrances, but rather, absorb the molecules that cause lingering odors. Even better, they also remove other airborne chemicals in the process, including ammonia, bacteria, formaldehyde, methane, microbes, mold, smoke, and, most importantly, volatile organic compounds (VOCs).

According to the owner of airCOAL®, "Skeptics by nature, we began scientific testing and confirmed with a VOC meter that 70% of gas molecules were in fact being captured within 4 hours by Bamboo Charcoal in a sealed container". Obviously, one would need a few of these pouches to clean a whole house, but they do maintain that each pouch is equivalent to 12 boxes of baking soda (in odor absorption potential).

This ability to remove VOCs makes bamboo charcoal ideal to use in new cars, to absorb the off gassing of plastics, and other chemical compounds, which create that new car smell. Anecdotal feedback on their website indicates the product works well for this function. Retailing for about $9 (CAD), it lasts for one year, and then can be recycled into your garden soil as a fertilizer. (www.aircoal.com)

BPA

Another xenoestrogen prevalent in modern life is Bisphenol A (BPA). BPA removes protective molecules that prevent genes from being turned on at the wrong time, or in the wrong tissue. And, many studies have found that BPA, like phthalates, interferes with hormones.

Animal tests indicate exposure to BPA in the womb raises the risk of certain cancers—especially cancer of the breast and prostate—hampers fertility, and could contribute to hyperactivity in children.

One human study has linked BPA to the development of asthma in children, while another showed reduced lung capacity in children exposed to BPA in the womb. This study found that "every 10-fold increase in the average maternal urinary BPA concentration had a marginal association with a 54.8% increase in the likelihood of the child wheezing. A 10-fold increase in the maternal urinary BPA concentration at 16 weeks of gestation was associated with a 4.27-fold increase in the likelihood of persistent wheezing". (3)

An animal study (done on mice) indicated that BPA also alters the function of mouse pancreatic cells (which produce insulin), suggesting the chemical may increase the risk of developing Type II diabetes. Another rodent study found that BPA led to increased growth, suggesting that the chemical might trigger obesity. No surprise there, since excess estrogen is already linked to obesity. In fact, a study from the University of Rochester found men with the highest level of phthalates in their bodies, had 3-inch wider waists than those with the lowest levels.

BPA is found in polycarbonate bottles (#7, including baby bottles, and home-delivery water bottles), microwave ovenware, eating utensils, shiny paper receipts, and plastic coatings for metal cans. Most cans are now lined with plastic, making canned goods one of our main sources of BPA ingestion. As well, both beer and soda cans are lined inside with a water-based polymer lining that contains BPA.

There is clear evidence BPA can leach into food, and drinks, from the lining of containers. One study demonstrated that eating canned soup for 5 days in a row increased urinary BPA concentration by more than 1000%, in comparison with eating soup made from fresh ingredients. Another study, confirming this, also found that BPA elevated blood pressure.

In this study, 60 participants (all over age 60), participated in the experiment three times. Each time, they were randomly given soymilk in either two glass bottles, two cans, or one can and one glass bottle. Following the consumption of canned soymilk, participant's urinary BPA concentration rose by up to 1,600%, compared with consumption of soymilk from glass bottles. The researchers were surprised to find an increase in blood pressure to accompany the increase in BPA, which, while not severe, was still statistically significant.

"A 5 mmHg increase in systolic blood pressure by drinking two canned beverages may cause clinically significant problems, particularly in patients with heart disease or hypertension," said study author Dr. Yun-Chul Hong of Seoul National University College of Medicine. (4)

It is considered a fact that a 20 mmHg increase in systolic blood pressure doubles the risk of cardiovascular disease. So it is unfortunate this study did not continue on to find out what increase in blood pressure occurred from 4 cans, or 6 cans, since it is not unusual for people to consume a number of canned beverages (along with canned food) on a daily basis.

TETRA-PAKS AND PET PLASTIC

Since industry has become aware of the widespread consumer knowledge of BPA, many plastic containers now advertise themselves as BPA-free. However, there are other plastic compounds which can also be dangerous, compounds not yet been fully identified, or which have not received the negative publicity that BPA has.

Two of the containers we most commonly use, found in both commercial grocery stores and health food stores, are PET, or PETE (Polyethylene terephthalate) bottles, and Tetra Paks. Coincidentally, the company that makes Tetra Pak (Tetra Laval) is also the producer of PET bottles, via their subsidiary SIDEL.

A wide variety of foods, including many organic ones, such as juice, milk, milk substitutes, soup, and wine, are packaged in Tetra Paks—one reason being these products do not require refrigeration.

However, it may be the advantages of purchasing organic foodstuffs, are negated by the packaging in which they come—if we use Tetra Paks.

Tetra Paks are made from paperboard, but in order to make it air and water proof, the paperboard has to be lined with aluminum coated in plastic. This plastic coating is a petroleum-derived, low-density polyethylene (LDPE).

PET (#1) plastic bottles are BPA-free, and are used for almost all bottled waters (except those in glass containers), as well as for juices, and soda. PET may well be BPA-free, but a recent German study has revealed these plastic bottles nonetheless leach xenoestrogens into the water they contain.

In this study, some snails were raised in water contained in PET plastic bottles, and others in water contained in glass bottles. Those snails raised in the plastic bottles produced about twice as many embryos as those raised in glass bottles. The scientists attributed this unnatural effect on the fertility of these snails, to xenoestrogens leached into the water from the PET plastic containers.

The authors of this German study, in their conclusion, also referred to other studies that supported their position: "In a recent study, Montuori et al. (2008) compared mineral waters bottled in glass and PET and detected significantly higher amounts of phthalates (DMP, DEP, DiBP, DBP, and DEHP) in plastic bottled water. The sum of studied compounds was thus 12 times higher in water from PET bottles compared to samples from glass bottles. Taken together, there is good analytical evidence for the migration of certain phthalates from PET food packaging materials, some of them well-known xenoestrogens." (Jobling et al. 1995)

This study also observed the metal antimony (used as a catalyst in plastic production) also leached into the water; and other earlier studies, also found antimony leached into water stored in PET containers. At this point, there is no information on the dangers of ingesting antimony (though industrial exposure is considered dangerous). As a side note, the leaching of antimony into water increases dramatically when the water is exposed to a hot environment for a lengthy period of time—so do not leave bottled water in the sun, or in a hot vehicle. (5)

Other studies, from this same German group, found Tetra Paks also showed xenoestrogens leaching into their contents, which they attributed to the plastic lining. Furthermore, the Tetra Paks in fact leached more xenoestrogens than the PET bottles, so, even though these containers do not contain BPA, they certainly do contain estrogen-mimicking chemicals. The researchers stated, "Though yet unidentified, these substances act as functionally active estrogens in vitro on the human estrogen receptor alpha and in vivo in a molluskan model". (6)

Here I should point out that acidic foods and liquids (like soda pop, fruit juice, alcohol, and tomatoes) will increase the amount of leaching far beyond what water will extract. And, in this study, they used mineral water, which is more alkaline than many foods. So, even though many plastics now proudly declare that they are "BPA-free", we should still choose glass containers over plastic, whenever possible.

TIPS FOR AVOIDING EXPOSURE TO XENOESTROGENS

- We can do our best to avoid xenoestrogen pesticides by purchasing mostly organic foods. Since dioxins, and organochlorine pesticides, build up in animal fat—increasing our exposure when we eat eggs, fatty meats, and milk-based products—we should also ensure our meat and dairy products are organic, whenever possible.

- Avoid shampoos, soaps, lotions, and other skin products containing members of the paraben family (butyl, ethyl, methyl, propyl), phenoxyethanol, red dye no.3, polyethylene glycol (PEG), and any chemicals that include the name dioxin.

- Avoid water bottled in plastic. Kleen Kanteen, and other brands, made from stainless steel, and Sigg (non-reactive, ceramic-coated interior) water bottles, are free of leaching chemicals, including BPA. Just add filtered tap water, or home-delivered spring water, and you avoid ingesting plastic molecules, and avoid adding more plastic to the environment.

- Do not cook food in plastic containers in a microwave. Rather, cook your food in, or on, a regular stove, using cast iron, surgical stainless steel, titanium, or glass cookware. Even if a plastic container says it is microwave safe, microwaving it will cause more of the chemicals in the plastic to leach into the food. If you must microwave (and I strongly suggest that you do not), always use a glass container.

- Avoid using plastic containers to store your food, and do not take hot liquids from Styrofoam (expanded polystyrene) containers.

- Use natural laundry detergents, and do not use dryer sheets, or fabric softener.

- Avoid air fresheners for home or car.

- Do not use chemical pesticides on your lawn and gardens.

- Only use feminine hygiene products made from organic, unbleached cotton.

- Use unbleached (or not chlorine bleached) toilet and tissue paper.

- Avoid commercial nail polish and solvent removers.

- Use natural birth control instead of birth control pills: the synthetic estrogen adds to the total estrogen load on the body, making it less able to cope with xenoestrogens.

- Avoid using and inhaling chemical glue, paint, and solvents.

- Try to use canned goods packaged in enamel-lined cans (available in health food stores).

- If you are buying conventional canned goods, avoid those which contain acidic substances (like tomatoes, and fruit and fruit juices), as they are more likely to leach plastic compounds into the foods. Choose those canned goods in glass, when available.

- Do not purchase acidic foods, and beverages, packaged in flexible (soft) plastic containers. Flexible plastic leaches easily even into water, but worse are alcohol (which is also a solvent), fruit, fruit juices, soda pop, tomatoes, and tomato juices.

- When using plastic containers, avoid heating them, or putting them through the dishwasher, as this will increase the amount of leaching that occurs. Use glass or ceramic containers instead, and look for products with code #2 (high density polyethylene), #4 (low density polyethylene), or #5 (polypropylene).

For more information on safely choosing and using plastics, search for "Smart Plastics Guide: Healthier Food Uses of Plastics", which is found at www.iatp.org.

For more information on the subject, the non-profit society, Environmental Working Group, is a place to find objective information on a wide variety of chemical contaminants in all areas of modern living (www.ewg.org).

PROTECTIVE NUTRIENTS

Now for some good news: there are certain dietary and nutritive measures we can take to both protect us from xenoestrogens and to help expel them from our bodies.

Methyl Donors

Certain nutrients have a protective function, when it comes to these hormone-disrupting chemicals. Of these, those that serve as "methyl-donors" are the most valuable. Methyl donors are involved in the metabolism of fats and DNA, and methylation of DNA can prevent the expression of damaging genes—including cancer genes.

Methyl-based nutrients are essential for liver detoxification pathways to function well. When the body has to cope with toxins difficult for the liver to remove—such as fat-soluble, or other relatively insoluble toxins—it joins these toxins to a methyl group, making them far easier to remove from the body.

Essentially, the methylation reaction makes toxins water-soluble. This allows the body to remove these compounds much more effectively, and, as well, neutralizes some of their toxic properties. These toxins include all of the heavy metals, as well as hundreds of other toxic chemicals, including xenoestrogens.

Folic acid and vitamin B-12 (methylcobalamin form) are the most well known methyl donors. We require a minimum of 1 mg of folic acid (in the superior form, known as methylfolate), and 100 mcg of B-12, daily, though it is safe to take much higher doses of B12 (up to 1000 mcg daily), without professional advice.

Other supplemental forms of methyl donors include DMAE (Dimethylaminoethanol), DMG (Dimethylglycine), TMG (Trimethylglycine), and SAMe (S-adenosylmethionine). Of these, if we had to choose one, simply for the function of methyl donation, the choice would be TMG. A recommended maintenance dose is 1 gram, 3 times daily, with a gradual doubling of that for more serious conditions. If you feel dizzy, nauseous, or get a headache, just reduce the amount: this can occur due to detoxification occurring too fast.

Genistein, a phytoestrogen derived from soy, also helps to methylate DNA. Other foods are also high in methyl donors, including garlic, onions, and beets—all considered detoxifiers in the natural health field. Beet juice is an easy and healthful way to get methyl donors into the body, and serves many other helpful functions as well (including blood-building, and vasodilation).

Chlorella

Chlorella, a fresh water algae rich in nutrients, is renowned for its powerful detoxifying abilities. Chlorella is high in RNA and DNA, which supports cellular repair, and it cleans the bowel, blood, and liver of toxins, and heavy metals. It is also one of the few substances which can remove pesticides from the body (including DDT, and PCBs). The dosage of chlorella ranges from 3 to 6 grams daily (with more being used therapeutically, for a short time).

As well, chlorella helps the body to remain alkaline, which is of critical importance to good health—much of the damage done by modern chemicals occurs because they are so acidifying to the body. If you are not sure about your acid/alkaline status, you can purchase pH strips from vitamin stores, and chart your levels.

Flax

Phytoestrogens, or plant estrogens, will occupy estrogen cell receptors—displacing excessive, or synthetic, estrogen—and, as a result, are sometimes referred to as anti-estrogens. One of the most protective phytoestrogens is a component of flax seeds called lignans. Five to ten grams of fresh ground (or pre-ground, but defatted) flax seed, daily, will displace strong, or synthetic, estrogens. Lignans will also block testosterone from breaking down into DHT, which causes swelling of the prostate. In one limited study (25 men), a high lignan intake reduced the rate of cancer cell growth in the prostate, and lowered PSA levels as well.

Flax is of course also a good source of fiber, and excess estrogen will bind to fiber. So, keeping fiber intake high, also helps to remove xenoestrogens from the body. This also prevents toxemia caused by constipation, where the body absorbs more toxins because they are stored too long in the bowel, instead of being evacuated regularly.

Friendly Flora

Friendly bacteria are also necessary to keep regular, and to keep the bowel clean, and free of toxins, but there is another advantage to one specific form of probiotic: bifidobacterium bifidus.

Estrogen is not active until it binds to a receptor. Therefore, the greater number of estrogen receptors you have in your breasts, uterine, and ovarian cells (in women), and prostatic cells (in men), the more susceptible you are to the effects of xenoestrogens. Butyrate—produced by the friendly bacteria, bifidobacterium bifidus, present in your large intestine—decreases the production of estrogen receptors. Thus, this strain of probiotic can help protect us from the damaging effects of many xenoestrogens.

Two other strains of probiotics help the body specifically excrete BPA. In an animal study, researchers evaluated bifidobacterium breve, and lactobacillus casei, to see if they could exert a protective effect against dietary exposure to BPA. In this study, rats receiving either of these two bacteria showed a clear advantage in clearing BPA from their bodies, since the amount of BPA excreted in their feces was significantly greater (2.4 times) than the control group. The study concluded, "These results suggest that bifidobacterium breve and lactobacillus casei reduced the intestinal absorption by facilitating the excretion of BPA, and that these probiotics may suppress the adverse effects of BPA on human health". (7)

So, look for high amounts of these specific strains when purchasing a probiotic product. And, ensure that you eat a good amount of fermented foods, which will help those species (as well as all your beneficial flora) thrive in your intestines. Another option is a spore-based probiotic, like LactoSpore (available from NutriStart, in Canada), which, like fermented foods, also encourages your indigenous good bacteria to colonize, while discouraging bad bacteria from growing.

LactoSpore is especially helpful for those who find other probiotic products to be disruptive, or unhelpful. Unlike most probiotics, Lactospore does not work by imposing colonies of specific strains on the digestive tract, on the assumption that one formulation is good for all people. Rather, it supports your unique microbiome, returning it to the healthful balance required for your body—not imposing other bacteria in ratios that may not be ideal for your system.

Ginger

Ginger is an amazing food/herb with many healthful properties, including improving digestion, reducing nausea, and stabilizing blood sugar levels. Ginger is also rich in antioxidants, and works as a powerful anti-inflammatory. In addition to this, ginger is an excellent detoxifier, and studies have shown it protects against the damaging effects of a number of chemical toxins.

One of the toxins that ginger protects against is lindane (the aforementioned xenoestrogenic neurotoxin), used as a pesticide, and in lice medication. Ginger was also shown to protect rats against the chemical bromobenzene (damages the liver), the cancer drug doxorubicin (damages the kidneys), and MSG (a neurotoxin). (8)

Glutathione

Glutathione is a master detoxifier, and part of your free radical defense system. It can help prevent the side effects of xenoestrogens, and works to detoxify the chemical contaminants we come into contact with, on a daily basis. The following substances are your best elevators of glutathione in the body. (Note that most supplemental forms of glutathione are ineffective, except for intravenous, sublingual, or liposomal forms.)

Vitamin C (500-1000 mg three times daily)
R-Alpha Lipoic Acid (100-200 mg three times daily)
N-acetyl cysteine (500 mg three times daily)
Milk Thistle (80% silymarin – 250 mg two times daily)
Whey Protein Isolate (15 to 25 gr, once or twice daily)
Liposomal Glutathione (250-500 mg daily)

All of these nutrients also support the liver, and its detoxification functions. Foods that support liver function include beets, celery, carrots, and parsley, along with the herbs dandelion (root), and burdock. As well, eating raw and fermented organic fruits and vegetables, in moderation, provides enzymes the body needs for digestion, and the elimination of toxins. (I say "in moderation" because too much raw food can actually be problematic for some digestive systems, and certain health conditions.)

Turmeric

As mentioned in the chapter on Radioprotective Supplements, most scientific studies done with turmeric, are based on using the isolated component, "curcumin"—considered its active element. However, as with many antioxidants, isolated compounds can also have pro-oxidant activities. This means isolated antioxidants can also produce free radicals, if not constrained by the checks and balances the other compounds (found in the whole food) provide. This is why we should always take a mixed variety of antioxidants in supplement form, and not high levels of just one, isolated, nutrient.

That being said, I will nonetheless refer to two studies that have shown curcumin to protect against xenoestrogen-induced cancer activity. However, we will assume that using the whole turmeric root (or powder), or supplements with standardized curcuminoid levels, will work even better at this function, than curcumin alone.

In one study, published in the journal Phytotherapy (2014), curcumin reversed BPA-induced cancer within cells exposed to the xenoestrogen. The researchers concluded, "Findings from this study could provide new insights into the molecular mechanisms by which BPA exerts its breast-cancer-promoting effect as well as its target intervention". (9)

In another study, curcumin suppressed phthalate-induced cancer growth in liver cells representative of the most common type of liver cancer, and, in live animal experiments, inhibited tumor growth and metastasis. They concluded, "Our results suggest that curcumin may be a potential antidote for phthalate-induced cancer progression". (10)

OTHER PROTECTIVE COMPOUNDS

- Three other compounds that effectively detoxify and eliminate excess, or synthetic estrogens, are indole-3-carbinol (I3C), diindoylmethane (DIM), and sulfurophane. All are available as supplements, or found naturally occurring in cruciferous vegetables (broccoli, Brussels sprouts, cabbage, cauliflower, kale, etc.—all best eaten sprouted, fermented, or cooked, to prevent thyroid inhibition).

■ Another substance, calcium d-glucarate, prevents the re-absorption of excreted estrogens. It is available in supplement form, and occurs in two foods particularly rich in calcium d-glucarate: apples and grapefruit (ideally organic).

■ The antioxidant compounds, polyphenols, found in green tea, and grape seed extract, also protect against estrogen-related cancers. (Remember, the benefits of green tea accrue at 3 to 5 cups per day).

SWEATING OUT XENOESTROGENS

A group of scientists released two studies looking at how we might use the xenoestrogen content of body fluids to help determine toxicity, and how sweating may be a useful way to eliminate these compounds from our bodies.

In one study, they examined BPA and noted, "There is incomplete understanding of BPA toxicokinetics, and there are no established interventions to eliminate this compound from the human body".

This study was designed to assess the relative concentration of BPA in three body fluids—blood, urine, and sweat—and to determine whether induced sweating may have the potential to help elimination BPA from the body. In 16 of 20 participants, BPA was found to varying degrees, in their blood, urine, and sweat. However, BPA was also found in sweat from some individuals who showed no BPA in their blood, or urine, samples.

This led the researchers to conclude that monitoring BPA exclusively through blood and/or urine testing may underestimate the total body burden of this toxin. Therefore, sweat analysis should be considered as an additional method for monitoring the accumulation of BPA in humans. They also confirmed that, "induced sweating appears to be a potential method for elimination of BPA". (11)

In the second study, they looked at different members of the xenoestrogen family: the phthalates. The scientists were well aware that "studies have demonstrated statistically significant exposure-disease relationships involving phthalates and toxicological studies have shown estrogenic effects in vitro". But, what they found lacking in medical literature, was an effective means to facilitate phthalate excretion.

Again, they collected blood, urine, and sweat, from 20 individuals, and analyzed for phthalate compounds. They found "all the patients had MEHP (mono-(2-ethylhexyl) phthalate) in their blood, sweat, and urine samples, suggesting widespread phthalate exposure".

And again, in some of the participants, one phthalate, DEHP (di (2-ethylhexl) phthalate) was found in sweat, but not in the blood samples, "suggesting the possibility of phthalate retention and bioaccumulation. On average, MEHP concentration in sweat was more than twice as high as urine levels". This led to the same conclusions as their BPA study: "Sweat analysis may be helpful in establishing the existence of accrued DEHP in the human body, and induced perspiration may be useful to facilitate elimination of some potentially toxic phthalate compounds." (12)

While sweating can be induced by vigorous exercise, and traditional steam saunas, the best detoxification technology is to use an infrared sauna (with "near" infrared being somewhat superior to "far" infrared). For those who cannot afford to purchase these saunas, they are often available at alternative medical clinics (or even some tanning salons) for rental by the hour. Making yourself sweat—via hydrotherapy, exercise, or sauna—both removes toxins and heavy metals, and improves nutrient circulation throughout the body.

To get the most out of a sauna one should ideally exercise for 10 to 20 minutes, and/or take a niacin pill (to the flush-point), before entering the sauna. Next to a sauna, the best external detoxifier is a bath containing 1 to 2 cups of sea salt and 1 to 2 cups of baking soda (also more effective with niacin taken beforehand). As well, drinking sufficient purified water is necessary for the elimination of toxins through the kidneys, and is especially important to do when using saunas.

Initially, when having a detox bath, the water should be very hot, in order to bring blood to the surface of the skin. This makes it easier for the salt and baking soda to draw toxins out through the skin. One can cool the water down a bit, if it is uncomfortably hot, but to have the best detoxification experience, you should not add any more hot water to the bath once you are in it.

As the water cools down (about 30 to 45 minutes later), the toxins are more easily drawn into the water via osmosis; the heat from the warmed body is pulled, along with the toxins, into the cooling water. Therefore, for maximum benefit, during a detox bath it is important that one let the water cool down before exiting the bath.

Also, for optimal efficiency, do not shower off after the bath but just towel dry. This type of bath ideally should be done in the evening, since one is usually very tired after taking a detox bath.

Endnotes

1. Steroids. 1999 May; 64(5):328-34; "Xenoestrogen interaction with human sex hormone-binding globulin (hSHBG)"; Déchaud H, et al.

2. Schecter, Arnold. "Intake of Dioxins and Related Compounds from Food in the US Population." Journal of Toxicology and Environmental Health, 2001

3. "Bisphenol A Exposure and the Development of Wheeze and Lung Function in Children Through Age 5 Years." Spanier et al., JAMA Pediatrics, published 6 October 2014

4. "Exposure to Bisphenol A from drinking canned beverage increases blood pressure." Yun-Chul Hong and Sanghyuk Bae, Hypertension, published online 8 December 2014

5. J Environ Health Sci Eng. 2014; 12: 133. "Effects of storage time and temperature on the antimony and some trace element release from polyethylene terephthalate (PET) into the bottled drinking water." Ebrahim Molaee Aghaee, et al.

6. Environmental Science and Pollution Research; May 2009, Volume 16, Issue 3, pp 278–286; "Endocrine disruptors in bottled mineral water: total estrogenic burden and migration from plastic bottles." Martin Wagner, Jörg Oehlmann.

7. Biosci Biotechnol Biochem. 2008 Jun; 72(6):1409-15. "Effect of probiotics, Bifidobacterium breve and Lactobacillus casei, on bisphenol A exposure in rats." Oishi K, et al.

8. "Protective effects of dietary ginger (Zingiber officinales Rosc.) on lindane-induced oxidative stress in rats." Rafat S. Ahmed, et al; Phytotherapy Research; Volume 22, Issue 7, pages 902–906, July 2008.

9. "Curcumin Modulates miR-19/PTEN/AKT/p53 Axis to Suppress Bisphenol A-induced MCF-7 Breast Cancer Cell Proliferation." Xiaoting Li, et al. Phytotherapy Research; Volume 28, Issue 10, pages 1553–1560, October 2014

10. J Agric Food Chem. 2015 Dec 9; 63(48):10388-98. "Curcumin Suppresses Phthalate-Induced Metastasis and the Proportion of Cancer Stem Cell (CSC)-like Cells via the Inhibition of AhR/ERK/SK1 Signaling in Hepatocellular Carcinoma." Tsai CF, et al.

11. J Environ Public Health. 2012; 2012:185731. "Human excretion of bisphenol A: blood, urine, and sweat (BUS) study." Genuis SJ, et al.

12. Scientific World Journal. 2012; 2012: 615068. "Human elimination of phthalate compounds: blood, urine, and sweat (BUS) study." Genuis SJ, et al.

PART THREE

ELECTROMAGNETIC POLLUTION

ELECTROSMOG

*"Electromagnetic pollution may be the most signifi-
cant form of pollution human activity has produced
in this century, all the more dangerous because it is an
invisible and insensible 'toxin'."*

Dr. Andrew Weil

I believe most of the things in modern life that kill us are invisible. In the past predators were the obvious danger, but now the closest analogy is the car, which, up until recently, was the leading cause of death until middle age (when cancer and heart disease take over). Now, as discussed in the chapter "Death by Medicine", prescription drugs have replaced car accidents as the leading cause of death, accompanied by other hidden dangers lurking in the hospital.

Many of the causes of cancer, heart disease, and other life-threatening ailments are also invisible: hidden in our foods (trans-fats, preservatives, acrylamide, radiation, and genetically modified organisms); cosmetics and body care products (hormone-disrupting and estrogen-mimicking chemicals); water (ammonia, chlorine, fluoride, water-borne parasites and pharmaceutical drug residues); air (smog, chemical fumes); and homes (flame-retardant chemicals, formaldehyde, and various molds).

WHAT IS ELECTROSMOG?

Another deadly invisible agent, paid little attention to in North America (though more so in Europe), is electromagnetic fields (EMFs). Any strong electrical current puts off a field that has—depending on whom you believe—either a small, or great, effect on the human organism. This type of field has been affecting humans since the dawn of widespread electricity. In fact, researcher Samuel Milhamemail believes the widespread diseases of the 20th century are directly linked to the advent of electricity. Now we have many more forms of these types of fields due to cell phone towers, wireless technology, and smart meters.

Depending on the energy output and frequency, electromagnetic waves are classified as either "ionizing radiation", or "non-ionizing radiation". Ionizing radiation comes from gamma rays (found in nuclear plants, and decaying radioactive material), X-rays, and those things we commonly think of as "radioactive". These rays produce enough photon energy to cause ionization (create positive and negative electrically charged atoms) by breaking the atomic bonds that hold cell molecules together.

Non-ionizing radiation (NIR) refers to those electromagnetic fields that have photon energies too weak to break the atomic bonds holding molecules together. They include ultraviolet radiation, infrared radiation, magnetic fields, and microwave and radio frequency fields.

Because even high intensity NIR cannot cause ionization in a biological system, conventional science maintains they cannot be responsible for damaging health in humans. Their position is, since the NIR cannot break molecular bonds in our cells, it cannot damage DNA, and therefore cannot contribute to cancer, or other degenerative diseases.

As we will see, this is not necessarily so. For one thing, NIR can produce other biological effects. By heating cells (remember, microwaves are used to cook things), altering chemical reactions, and/or inducing electrical currents in tissues and cells, NIR can have a significant negative impact on our health.

EMF, EMR & RF

"Electromagnetic waves at low frequencies are referred to as 'electromagnetic fields' and those at very high frequencies are called 'electromagnetic radiations'."—World Health Organization: Electromagnetic Fields and Public Health.

What I will be discussing in this, and the following related chapters, is non-ionizing radiation. NIR is divided into three subcategories.

Electromagnetic fields (**EMFs**) refer to the energy waves radiated by conventional electronic devices, and household wiring. This is a different frequency from microwaves, which comprise another invisible field found everywhere in cities—due to cell phone towers. These frequencies are referred to as electro-magnetic radiation (**EMR**), while Wi-Fi and smart meters are categorized as radio frequencies (**RF**). For the sake of convenience, I will use the term electromagnetic pollution, or electrosmog, when generalizing.

HOW CAN THESE FIELDS BE DANGEROUS?

Our bodies are a complex communication network, where cells and organs exchange data continuously. This form of communication is considered bio-electrical, and just as a TV or radio antenna signal can be disrupted by external electronic pulses (producing static or noise), so our internal biochemical signals can be disrupted by too much exposure to this kind of electromagnetic pollution.

An important part of our internal bio-electrical communication system is based on the permeability of our cell membranes. When the cell wall is permeable, it allows nutrients into, and removes toxins out of, the cell. These cells are sensitive to even low-level electromagnetic interference, which (like exposure to chemical toxins and heavy metals) severely reduces the permeability of the cell.

Some scientists also believe electromagnetic pollution can interfere with the correct functioning of brain waves, and the physical body. So much so, that neurological problems (like dementia), and physiological problems (like fibromyalgia and chronic fatigue syndrome), can be linked to excessive electrosmog exposure. There are also recent scientific implications that electromagnetic pollution—while it may not directly damage DNA—can impede the body's ability to repair DNA, which alone could contribute to the development of cancer, and premature aging.

HEALTH ISSUES LINKED TO EMFS

I recall a fellow with the beginnings of Parkinson's disease who used to frequent a vitamin store in which I worked. He would drive to the store without issue, but within 15 minutes of being exposed to the fluorescent lights, the old ballasts (which put out very high EMFs), and the high electromagnetic frequencies being put off by all the coolers, his hands would shake so badly, the vitamin bottle he was holding would sound like a rattle. People like him, with those types of neurological disorders, are our "canaries in the coal mines", and are the first to show the most symptoms from exposure to strong electromagnetic fields.

One thing we know for sure about EMFs (based on clinical studies), is they deplete melatonin levels. Low melatonin levels are linked to poor sleep patterns, immune malfunction, and certain types of cancer. So, while EMFs may not directly cause cancer by damaging DNA, they can indirectly contribute to cancer by drastically lowering melatonin levels in the body.

Aside from EMFs emitted from conventional electrical wiring, and devices, one unexpected source of EMFs is the cars we drive. Newer cars—ones that have computers operating in the engines—emit far more EMFs than old cars, which are strictly mechanical.

New studies have indicated that electric, and hybrid, cars can be an even higher source of EMFs than the newer gasoline powered vehicles. Due to the location of the battery, hybrid cars produced the highest EMF readings in the back right seat—and the electromagnetic fields grow in strength with increased speed, peaking at around 80 km/h.

"Passengers inside an Electric Vehicle could be exposed to Magnetic Fields of considerable strength when compared with conventional vehicles or to other daily exposures (at home, in the office, in the street, etc)." (Pablo Moreno-Torres Concha, et al. Passenger Exposure to Magnetic Fields due to the Batteries of an Electric Vehicle. IEEE Transactions on Vehicular Technology. 65(6):4564-4571. Jun 2016)

Ailments linked to EMF exposure, and sensitivity, include, chronic fatigue syndrome, fibromyalgia, anxiety, breathing difficulties, depression, dizziness, headaches, heart palpitations, tinnitus, ADD/ADHD, sleep disorders, lowered immune function, and neurological conditions, including MS, ALS, and numbness, tingling, and tremors.

ELECTROMAGNETIC HYPERSENSITIVITY

The Women's College Hospital, in Toronto, is one of the only medical organizations to agree with the premise that EMFs are deleterious. This hospital released a statement identifying certain symptoms as being indicative of a condition they call Electro-Magnetic Hypersensitivity, or EMS. The main symptoms include disrupted sleep, headaches, nausea, dizziness, heart palpitations, memory problems, and skin rashes.

The medical director of the hospital's Environmental Health Clinic, Dr. Riina Bray, stated, "We need to create more awareness about this condition. Health-care practitioners need to better understand EMS so they can help their patients prevent and manage their symptoms. The public needs to know how to protect themselves from the broad range of health impacts electromagnetic fields have on their minds and bodies".

Unfortunately, since they are the only medical professionals who believe electromagnetic hypersensitivity is a real issue, they are swamped with applicants to their clinic—where it can take up to 9 months to get an appointment to be diagnosed for EMS.

In 2001, "Electrical Hypersensitivity" was recognized as a medical condition by the Swedish government. They estimated that just over 3% of their population was severely affected by this condition. I would suggest this 3% represents only the tip of the iceberg, and that many more of us are affected by EMFs. For most people, the constant exposure will slowly grind away at their health, not being identified until a full-blown disease finally manifests. At which point, they will only be told they have heart failure, diabetes, or cancer, and the link between EMFs and their ailment will never be made.

CELL PHONE TOWERS

Many people have by now, at least heard the theory that prolonged cell phone use has been associated with brain cancer. However, most people are still unaware that other sources of electromagnetic radiation can also dramatically increase cancer risk, including the towers cell phones depend on.

Studies, sponsored by the telecommunication industry, and accepted by the government, have promoted the idea that current EMR exposure levels are safe, and so, both individuals, and the medical profession, have ignored any potential dangers.

However, consider that North American governments receive huge tax revenues from the telecom industry, which encourages them not to be too critical of the flawed safety studies received from the foxes guarding the chicken coop.

Meanwhile, studies from non-industry supported scientific groups tell another story. These studies reveal the EMR from telecom towers, and antennas, seriously alter the body's cellular communication processes—potentially leading to cancer and other diseases. Since new cell phone towers are being constructed all the time, the amount of radiation exposure is practically doubling every year. Currently, the average city-dweller can have anywhere between 30 to 100 microwave towers within a 4-mile radius of their home.

Cell phone towers emit high-frequency electromagnetic waves (microwaves) that have been clearly linked to cancer development. For example, one German study reported that living within 1300 feet of two microwave towers, over ten years, triples cancer risk. Other studies from Australia, the UK, and Italy, revealed significant increases in leukemia among people who live near such towers. ("The Influence of Being Physically Near to a Cell Phone Transmission Mast on the Incidence of Cancer." Horst Eger, et al.; Published in Umwelt·Medizin·Gesellschaft 17, 4 2004)

My interest in discovering the true dangers of electromagnetic pollution began years ago, when I met some people who were living on a hill parallel to a bank of newly installed cell phone antennas. At that time, when such antennas were still uncommon, these people literally had to line their bedrooms with tinfoil, in order to sleep. (Mylar is now more commonly used to block out such frequencies.)

More recently, I have observed a friend of mine, hypersensitive to electromagnetic pollution, who immediately feels a myriad of severely unpleasant symptoms, when she gets too close to an array of cell phone antennas. Her breathing becomes constricted, she all of a sudden feels extremely drained, gets heart palpitations, her throat feels like it is closing off, and a general feeling of doom is experienced.

I have witnessed this in circumstances even when we had no idea there were cell phone antennas in the vicinity. Then, when we drove around the corner, we observed a large group of them. And, always, as we drive away from these antenna arrays, her symptoms abate.

People like her represent more of the "canaries", and, instead of being discounted as hypochondriacs, or paranoiacs, we should realize they are our early warning system. Even though most of us do not feel the obvious effects of these fields, electromagnetic pollution is nonetheless working insidiously to compromise our long-term health.

WI-FI

Cell phone towers are not the only source of electromagnetic pollution we are exposed to constantly. Wireless networking technology (Wi-Fi) connects electronic devices to wireless computer networks, using high-frequency radio waves. This form of electromagnetic pollution—emitted by Wi-Fi routers, baby monitors, and cordless phones—is also linked to cancer, along with other health problems. Unfortunately, more and more devices are now designed to use Wi-Fi, including all types of computers, video-game consoles, smart-phones, digital cameras, and digital audio players.

Unlike TV, and standard radio signals, Wi-Fi signals are powerful enough to penetrate concrete walls, and are designed to extend the frequency over a wide distance. If you have ever looked up the options for wireless links on your computer, you will find a list of often up to 30 options. Those are all wireless signals (coming from neighbors, and local businesses) which are running through your house—and body.

When industry does a test, they expose rats to a signal, for a limited time, and conclude it is safe. But, do they expose them to 30 overlapping Wi-Fi signals, slap on a bunch of microwave (cellphone) signals, and throw in the 20 RF signals from your neighbors' smart meters? I think not. Like with pesticide studies, every element is be tested alone, but no one does compounding tests to determine the effects of the total load, from all sources.

Some have gone so far as to state that, "Having a digital wireless device in your home, office, or school is like having a mini-base station (cell tower) indoors with you".—G. Blackwell, PhD (Advisor to www.wiredchild.org, a website devoted to "protecting our children from wireless technology".)

Wi-Fi is everywhere now, including homes, schools, offices,

hotels, airports, libraries, hospitals, and many public buildings. Just about every coffee shop, and retail store, boasts free wireless, many towns are bragging about free wireless for visitors, and the cable/internet companies are offering free wireless all over cities. As a result, we are more and more being blanketed in a sea of electrosmog. And, on top of that, the Canadian federal government has the wonderful idea of putting Wi-Fi into all the national parks. Lord help you if you are hypersensitive to EMFs; such people have no option but to relocate to the remote countryside.

Like all electromagnetic pollution, Wi-Fi radiation penetrates the body, affecting cell membranes, over time lessening the ability of cells to function properly. Wi-Fi exposure is linked to a wide range of symptoms, including anxiety, depression, fatigue, headaches, high blood pressure, hyperactivity, insomnia, fibromyalgia, infertility, irregular heartbeat, leukemia, nausea, poor concentration, stress, tinnitus, and weakened immune system.

WI-FI AND MERCURY

There are now more and more studies being done to determine the effects of Wi-Fi on biological organisms. One recent study clearly confirms it is having an effect on us, and it is a seriously bad effect.

For those who still have dental amalgam fillings, there is always concern that some mercury is leaching into the body, leading to potential health problems. Given that dental amalgam is composed of about 50% elemental mercury, this is no small concern.

Mercury, when released from dental fillings, can cross the blood brain barrier, affecting the central nervous system, and leading to severe immunological, neurological, and/or psychological, problems.

Recently a group of Brazilian scientists had the idea to "evaluate the effect of exposure to Wi-Fi signals on mercury release from amalgam restorations". The researchers gathered 20 teeth—which had been extracted at dental offices—filled them with amalgams (following standard dental protocols), and then stored the teeth in a saline solution, at body temperature, for 14 days. (They chose a 14 day timeframe because research indicates the highest amount of mercury discharges from fillings during the first 2 weeks after dental restorations are done.)

Following this, the tooth samples were put into tubes filled with artificial saliva, to mimic conditions in the human mouth. Then the teeth were divided into two groups: a control group and a group exposed to radiofrequency radiation, emitted from standard Wi-Fi devices, at 2.4 GHz for 20 minutes. The distance between the Wi-Fi router and the samples was 30 cm, and the router was exchanging data with a laptop computer placed 20 meters away from the router.

Results revealed the concentration of mercury in the Wi-Fi group to be roughly twice that of the control group. This led the researchers to conclude, "Exposure of patients with amalgam restorations to radiofrequency radiation emitted from conventional Wi-Fi devices can increase mercury release from amalgam restorations". (J Environ Health Sci Eng. 2016; 14: 12. "Effect of radiofrequency radiation from Wi-Fi devices on mercury release from amalgam restorations." Maryam Paknahad, et al.)

If this were not bad enough, consider also that mercury (along with other heavy metals) in the blood acts as an antenna, picking up more frequencies from all forms of electrosmog, and making us even more susceptible to their ill effects.

More information on the intrusion of wireless technologies into our lives, and what we can do about it, can be found at www.citizens-forsafetechnology.org.

SMART METERS

My aforementioned friend (hypersensitive to electrosmog) found her health rapidly deteriorating when her apartment building switched over to smart meters. Unfortunately for her, all twelve meters for the floor she was on, were in the electrical room on the other side of her kitchen. After the meters were installed she started to experience heart palpitations, shortness of breath, severe vertigo, and viral symptoms—ultimately forcing her to move.

And, of course, in the electrical room on the floor below, were another 12 smart meters, as well on each floor below that—as will be the case in any apartment building.

If you live in an apartment building, or condo, find out where the smart meters are gathered. If meters are adjacent to one of your walls, your apartment will be awash in high radio frequencies. You will definitely want to shield that wall with something, like foil-covered Mylar, or metal screening. Any meter installed inside the building (especially in the basement), will put out a stronger signal than one installed outside of the building, as it has to go through ceilings, floors and/or walls.

The way smart meters are determined to be safe (by industry) is by taking the short, strong bursts of radio waves they send out sporadically, and averaging that over the whole day—including the time that they are not transmitting. This average then looks like a low level of RF, when in fact that is just a numbers trick.

Some of the symptoms associated with radio frequencies emitted by smart meters include arrhythmia, dizziness, headaches, inflammation, irritability, short-term memory loss, mental fog, and sleep disturbance. In 2011, the WHO's International Agency for Research on Cancer classified wireless smart meter radiation as a 2B possible carcinogen for humans.

For a look at the science on smart meters and other forms of electromagnetic pollution visit, www.radiationresearch.org, or www.smartmeterharm.org

MORE EVIDENCE

The David Suzuki Foundation recommends people concerned about EMF pollution consult with the BioInitiative Report, for all the science related to damage done by these technologies. The BioInitiative Report was produced by 29 independent scientists, and health experts, from around the world, and covers all possible risks from wireless technologies, and electromagnetic fields. This report is freely available at www.bioinitiative.org.

The 2012 version of the BioInitiative Report covers about 1800 new studies, reporting adverse health effects of electromagnetic fields (power lines, electrical wiring, appliances, and hand-held devices), and wireless technologies (cell and cordless phones, cell towers, Wi-Fi, wireless routers, baby monitors, surveillance systems, wireless utility meters, etc.).

Subjects include "brain tumor risks from cell phones, damage to DNA and genes, effects on memory, learning, behavior, and attention, sleep disruption, cancer and neurological diseases like Alzheimer's disease, effects on sperm and miscarriage (fertility and reproduction), effects of wireless on the brain development of the fetus and infant, and effects of wireless classrooms on children and adolescents".

Following are some conclusions found in these 1800 new studies. Reports of, "abnormal gene transcription; genotoxicity and single-and double-strand DNA damage; stress proteins because of the fractal RF-antenna like nature of DNA; chromatin condensation and loss of DNA repair capacity in human stem cells; reduction in free-radical scavengers—particularly melatonin; neurotoxicity in humans and animals, carcinogenicity in humans; serious impacts on human and animal sperm morphology and function; effects on off-spring behavior; and effects on brain and cranial bone development in the offspring of animals that are exposed to cell phone radiation during pregnancy".

Not a pretty picture, and note they have indicated a mechanism whereby non-ionizing radiation appears to actually cause DNA damage. "Because of the fractal RF-antenna like nature of DNA," which appears to be a more recent discovery, they claim "loss of DNA repair capacity in human stem cells".

DNA is constantly being subjected to free radical damage from simply being alive, and our longevity is, in part, predicated on our ability to repair damaged DNA. Simply by inhibiting the body's ability to repair DNA, we have a scientifically valid mechanism by which these fields can lead to cancer, and other diseases.

STILL MORE EVIDENCE

Lest you still doubt the scientific veracity of what I have been writing about, this more recent material ought to be convincing.

In 2015, 190 scientists from 39 nations submitted an appeal to the United Nations, UN member states, and the World Health Organization. In this appeal, they requested more protective exposure guidelines for EMF and wireless technology, based on increasing evidence of risk to those exposed to this form of electromagnetic pollution.

Between them, this group of scientists has collectively published over 2,000 peer-reviewed papers on the biological and/or health effects of non-ionizing radiation (part of the EMF spectrum that includes Radio Frequency radiation, used for wireless communications).

This "International EMF Scientist Appeal" requested the Secretary General, and UN affiliated bodies, encourage precautionary measures to limit EMF exposures, and to educate the public about the health risks, especially to children and pregnant women.

One of the scientists, Martin Blank, PhD, of Columbia University, stated, "International exposure guidelines for electromagnetic fields must be strengthened to reflect the reality of their impact on our bodies, especially on our DNA. The time to deal with the harmful biological and health effects is long overdue. We must reduce exposure by establishing more protective guidelines".

They furthermore asked the UN to strengthen its advisories on EMF risks for humans, and to also examine the possible effect of EMF exposure to wildlife, and other living organisms, via the UN Environmental Program.

Another member of this group, Joel Moskowitz, PhD, of University of California, Berkeley, said, "ICNIRP guidelines set exposure standards for high-intensity, short-term, tissue-heating thresholds. These do not protect us from the low-intensity, chronic exposures common today. Scientists signing the Appeal request that the UN and member nations protect the global human population and wildlife from EMF exposures". (www.emfscientist.org)

BEES

Speaking of wildlife, like many creatures in the animal kingdom (such as birds, bats, and insects), bees also rely on the Earth's magnetic field and high frequency electromagnetic energy, for orientation, navigation, and communication. Because these creatures transmit, and receive, on certain frequencies, if there is too much interference or disruption occurring, it threatens their survival. Manmade electromagnetic fields—especially Wi-Fi and cell phone towers—are jamming and disrupting the bees' communication channels, disturbing their natural orientation and navigation mechanisms.

Renowned whistleblower George Carlo, a former insider from the mobile phone industry, who went public to expose the dangers of wireless, had this to say, in June 2007. "When the bee story first broke it was based on a German study that showed information-carrying radio waves disrupted the ability of bees to make it back to their hives….the mobile phone industry was caught off guard by the widespread media attention the story garnered…they conscripted scientists from a number of universities to begin going public with other explanations…viruses, bacteria, pesticides, etc."

The thing is, colony collapse disorder, as it is now known, occurred simultaneously on four continents within a very short period of time. If the reasons for this were chemical, or biological, there would have been a pattern to observe—much in the same way an epidemic spreads—but this is not the case: the situation struck all of the continents at roughly the same time. The rise of cell phone towers meets this criterion.

CANADIAN CONDEMNATION

Also in 2015, closer to home, The Canadian Medical Association Journal published a scathing condemnation of Health Canada's safety guidelines for cell phones and Wi-Fi.

The CMAJ interviewed a number of international experts on radiation and cancer, who convinced them the microwave levels allowed in Canadian classrooms, homes, and workplaces, are "a disaster to public health". This article quoted one scientist who said that, given the overwhelming evidence that wireless radiation is harmful, staff at Health Canada were either "unwilling or not competent enough to make evaluation of the current literature".

One cancer specialist, interviewed for this CMAJ article, maintained Canada's safety guidelines for wireless radiation need to be "urgently revised", due to an obvious cancer risk.

As this highly critical article also pointed out, the man who wrote Health Canada's safety code for wireless technologies, James McNamee, has in the past co-authored academic papers with scientists who openly accept payments from the wireless industry.

"That Canada's wireless safety code is out of date and mired in conflict of interest is no longer a question, it's a fact," said Frank Clegg, CEO of Canadians for Safe Technology. (www.c4st.org)

GREEN FASCISM

When you tell people (especially those in positions of authority) you do not want cell phone towers in your neighborhood, you don't want your children exposed to Wi-Fi in their schools, and you don't want a smart meter in your home, most regard you as paranoid and delusional. In our current culture, anything that interferes with commerce, convenience, and "business-as-usual", is suspect.

Like most of you, I love our planet, and believe we are fast destroying it. I personally think that debating global warming is a brilliant piece of sleight-of-hand by business. We used to call it pollution, and pollution was clearly bad. Now they have us debating global warming, while we continue to ravage the land, and foul the oceans, worse than ever. But, when government decides to tell you what you can and can't do, based on what they feel is best for you, and for the "future of the children," we have entered into what the British call the "nanny state".

Those in favor of this style of governing will cite tobacco regulations as an example of this being a reasonable approach, and, if we were able to actually trust the government, this might be a valid argument. However, the fact is, government, like science, has been co-opted by business.

There was a time when the medical profession encouraged smoking as a safe and healthy pastime. The government of America at that time, ensured soldiers at war were provided with tobacco, both for the benefits it offered for dealing with intense levels of stress, and for the handy pocket reminder of the home and freedom they were fighting for.

Now we have medical and government officials telling us that EMR from cell phone towers, wireless networks, etc., are safe enough to expose our children to. The level of concern from those, supposedly, protecting our health, is so low they often accomplish just the opposite.

I know of an array of cell phone antennas put on top of a government-owned apartment building—one designed to provide low-cost housing for seniors and the disabled—just to provide a little extra money to government coffers. There was no consideration given to how this might affect those (already weakened) individuals living there, who would be among the most susceptible to problems caused by, or associated with, EMR exposure.

Schools refuse to allow parents to prevent them from installing wireless networks—not at all concerned about exposing undeveloped

K.W. PETERS

brains to constant electro-magnetic fields. Then, school officials want the parents to put the children affected by this on drugs, to reduce the ensuing hyperactivity: a classic "Catch-22" situation.

"GREEN" FOR WHOM?

Currently, the business/government model has acquired a new paradigm to use in its manipulation of the public. They now have the "green" movement—easily co-opted, since it is a meme which engenders extreme emotions. Since most of us want to save the planet, obviously anything green must be good. And, if it is good, and we are too slow to immediately do what is "right", then sometimes the government just has to step in and make us do what they know is best. They know it is best because a lobbyist told them so, and provided them with the "evidence" they need, for the press releases.

GREEN BULBS AND SMART METERS

Two examples of this approach are compact fluorescent (or "green") light bulbs, and "smart meters" for recording electrical usage. The "green" bulbs save energy; that is their claim to fame and their one advantage. However, for those of us in the temperate to cold zones, the energy saved from the light bulb will have to be replaced with an identical thermal unit of energy, acquired from conventional heating sources. So the green light bulb is really only of value, from an energy perspective, in warm and hot areas, and in the summer for the rest of us. However, even this slight energy advantage is outweighed by the dangers they pose.

There are three serious problems with these bulbs. First, they put out high levels of ultraviolet radiation—enough to damage the skin if you sit too close to them—unless they are "shielded", which appears as a cover over the familiar spiral shape.

Second, these bulbs also emit huge amounts of EMFs, which tend to have the strongest negative effect on people already ill: those with compromised immune systems, neurological disorders, or electro-magnetic sensitivities.

IS MERCURY NOW "GREEN"?

Finally, to add insult to injury, if these green bulbs break, they release toxic amounts of mercury, and one needs to follow hazardous material clean-up protocols. Mercury is not very green is it? Yet someone decided for you that saving energy outweighs dumping more mercury into the environment—because ultimately, a lot of these bulbs are headed for the landfill. They decided this, and then they mandated it, so that incandescent bulbs have been outlawed, at the higher-wattage levels, and eventually all are to be outlawed (varying somewhat based on where you live). General Electric lobbyists started this ball rolling in the U.S., and Canada followed suit, like a good lapdog.

The mercury cleanup protocol for broken CFL bulbs has been tested, and revised, by the Maine State government, and I will include a summary of their suggested protocol at the end of this chapter. Personally, I would suggest exclusively using incandescent or LED lights.

"SMART" FOR WHOM?

The so-called "smart meters" are a great cost saver for the electric company—in part because they can lay off many workers who used to do the job of collecting data from each home—but many people are worried about yet another electromagnetic field running through their homes 24/7.

Did we have a choice in this matter? No. These meters have been installed in almost every home, except for a few homeowners that successfully resisted (no small feat), and now are allowed to pay a monthly fee to keep their old meters. As usual, those who support the party line simply mock those who are concerned, and imply that they are paranoid and non-scientific. After all, since they have hijacked the word "smart" if you disagree, well, then you must be the opposite of smart.

Since science is now a tool of industry, it will prove for you whatever outcome you require to further your business interests. These scientists-for-hire are like the doctors who said smoking was safe until the mid-1970s. The wireless industry is like the tobacco companies who will suppress data until it is no longer possible—then will pay out the class-action lawsuits filed against them, comprising a far lower sum of money than the profits they will make as this game plays out.

In some American states, the government has finally given people the right to have their old style meters back, due to claims of ill health, and unexplained electrical fires. We can hope this option will, at some point, be available to those of us in Canada, as well.

FREEDOM OF CHOICE

So where does individual freedom of choice come in, and to what point are you comfortable with the government telling you what is good for you, and that you have no options? After all, their track record is not that good if we look at history: our government is still paying reparations and making apologies to cultures we abused in the past. In fact, if we are to look to history, we can see that, in hindsight, governments are never fully trustworthy, as the best interests they have at heart are seldom those of its average citizens.

Now that the green movement has been partially taken over by industry, it is used as a mandate to push forward profit-making agendas—without anyone actually looking at the full picture, or the possible downsides to these new technologies. Therefore, it is critical we continue to question authority, and demand from our politicians the right to freedom of choice.

TESTING

Tracking these damaging frequencies is impossible without using a meter that tests for EMFs (electromagnetic frequencies), EMR (cell phones and cell towers), and RF frequencies (Wi-Fi, smart meters). These devices can be purchased through many companies found on the internet (www.lessemf.com, and www.slt.com, being two of the better ones). If you have health concerns that are not responding to conventional approaches, I suggest you purchase a testing meter. They are also rather interesting play with, and you may find the results quite surprising. (EMF meter reviews available at www.electricsense.com.)

Simple Gauss meters that check only for EMFs are relatively inexpensive (as little as $40 US), but since some of the meters that test for EMR and RF pollution can be quite expensive ($400 and up), there is also the option of hiring a professional to test your house, or workspace. Such people are available in most cities now, as more and more of us become aware of the current dangers (pun intended). Some of these technicians will also help plan new homes so that the dangers can be addressed before the houses are even built. (Find a list of consultants where you live at www.electricsense.com.)

As a rough reference range, one professional recommends readings should be less than the following values, in areas where people spend hours daily: 1 milliGauss for power frequency magnetic fields; 5 V/m for power frequency electric fields; 40 GS units for dirty electricity; 0.01 microW/cm2 for wireless radiation.

This data on electrosmog—along with the following chapter on cell phones—can be disturbing, but rest assured, I will follow up with chapters on coping strategies for dealing with these new forms of toxins.

COMPACT FLUORESCENT BULB CLEAN-UP

Most major retailers that sell CFBs offer free recycling collection for unbroken bulbs. As well, there is a recycle organization in most of the Canadian provinces (and a few US states), that take these bulbs for recycling, even if they are broken— provided that they are in a sealed plastic bag, or sealed glass container. (www.lightrecycle.ca)

The Maine State Government (providing the most thorough clean-up protocol I could find) recommends the following clean-up and disposal guidelines.

- Wear disposable gloves and before cleanup, vent the room— opening at least one window. Stay out of the room for at least 15 minutes after the breakage occurs. Ideally wear a surgical-style disposable facemask while doing the clean-up process, or at least breathe as little as possible during this time.

- If you have central forced air heating, or an air conditioning system, shut them off during the process.

- When cleaning up a broken bulb on a hard surface, carefully scoop up the glass fragments and powder using stiff paper or cardboard, and place them in a glass jar with a metal lid (such as a canning jar), or in a sealed thick plastic bag. Then use sticky tape, such as duct or packing tape, to pick up any remaining small glass fragments and powder, and put that into the container as well.

- Wipe the area clean with damp paper towels, or disposable wet wipes, and place those in the glass jar or plastic bag.

- Do not use a vacuum, or broom, to clean up the broken bulb on the hard surfaces, as that can cause the mercury powder to become airborne.

- When cleaning up a broken bulb on carpet or rug, carefully pick up glass fragments and place them in a glass jar with metal lid, or in a thick plastic bag. Use sticky tape to pick up any remaining small glass fragments and powder.

- Carpet or rugs may need vacuuming after all visible materials are removed. If so, vacuum area where the bulb was broken, wearing a mask, and ensuring there is airflow through the room. Then remove the vacuum bag (or empty and thoroughly wipe the canister), and put the bag or vacuum debris in the glass jar, or thick plastic bag.

- Immediately place the cleanup materials and broken bulb, in a sealed container, outside the building, until you are ready to dispose of it at a recycling center.

- Wash your hands, and any exposed areas, after removing gloves and disposing of the jars, or plastic bags, containing clean-up materials.

- Any future cleaning of carpets or rugs should be done while venting the room, both during and after vacuuming. For at least the next few times you vacuum, shut off the central forced-air heating, or air conditioning system, and open a window prior to vacuuming. Keep the central heating/air conditioning system shut off, and the window open, for at least 15 minutes after vacuuming is completed.

CELL PHONE RADIATION

"Brain tumors now account for more deaths among children and those under 40 than any other cancer."
www.braintumourresearch.org

We do love to talk, especially on the phone, with children and teens often having marathon conversations. Unfortunately, young people are the most susceptible to damage from cell phone radiation, as their skull bones are thinner than those of adults. To make matters worse, I recently discovered the average age for young people getting their first cell phone (or smart phone) is about 10 years old. Which of course, being an average, means that some kids are receiving these units at an even younger age. It is a good thing then, that texting has become a major way of communicating through these devices.

In this, and the following material, I primarily use the term cell phone, rather than smart phone, since the majority of the earlier studies were done when most people only had cell phones. But, since a smart phone is essentially a cell phone on steroids (requiring, and emitting, stronger electromagnetic fields than cell phones), you can assume the facts described below are even worse when applied to smart phones.

HEALTH RISKS

In 2009, the journal Pathophysiology published an overview of 15 studies (covering 6 countries) on the effects of electro-magnetic fields (EMFs), and radio frequency radiation (RF), on health. The editorial conclusion was not good: "Overall, the scientific evidence shows that the risk to health is significant and that to deny it is like being in free-fall and thinking 'so far, so good.'"

The response from those who safeguard our health in Canada was, sadly, predictable: "Health Canada currently sees no scientific reason to consider the use of cell phones as unsafe. There is no convincing evidence of increased risk of disease from exposure to radio frequency electromagnetic fields from cell phones."

Meanwhile, Martin Blank of Columbia University (editor of the report in Pathophysiology), took a different view: "Health Canada must realize that its obligation to protect the health of its citizens requires that they alert them to the implications of the scientific findings, so that they may take precautionary measures on their own."

Unfortunately, as mentioned earlier, the main health that Health Canada is concerned with is the health of business. While they can argue that most of the available science on the subject shows little risk, as mentioned earlier, most of this "science" was funded by telecom companies.

Currently, even as more independent science is swinging in the opposite direction, the majority of medical associations, including the American Cancer Society, the National Cancer Institute, the FDA, and the Canadian Medical Association, have all maintained that cell phones are totally safe.

CELL PHONES CLEARLY AFFECT THE BRAIN

In 2013, The Journal of the American Medical Association published a solid scientific study, proving beyond any doubt, "the human brain is sensitive to the electromagnetic radiation emitted by cell phones."

In this study, they used brain scans, which demonstrated that, after nearly an hour of exposure to cell phone radiation, there was an acceleration of activity in the section of the brain located closest to the antenna of the phone. What these brain scans measured was brain glucose metabolism—an indicator of brain activity.

The scientists involved made it clear they did not know if this increased activity was actually harmful to health. But the leader of the study, Dr. Volkow, did at least offer an opinion: "It also highlights the importance of doing studies to address the question of whether there are, or are not, long-lasting consequences of repeated stimulation, of getting exposed over five, 10 or 15 years."

The brain scans showed a 7% increase in brain activity in the area nearest the antenna, and while 7% may not look like much, the scientists considered it "statistically significant". This increased brain activity was not associated with the heat from the phone, since the activity occurred closer to the location of the antenna, rather than where the phone touched the head.

While this study may seem tame, and offer no cause for worry, it has two strong points. The first is that there is no debate in the scientific community about its validity. The second is that, up until now, the main argument of science (as to the safety of cell phones) is there is no known mechanism that can explain how cell phone frequencies could cause cancer.

Since scientists serving the telecom industry maintain cell phones do not have any effect on the human organism at all, the important thing this study shows is that they indeed do *something*—and that *something* may be a mechanism by which we can finally explain some of the dangers of cell phone use.

As mentioned before, radio frequency waves emitted by cell phones consist of "non-ionizing" radiation. This type of radiation is considered too weak to break chemical bonds in the cells, or to cause the DNA damage associated with cancer. However, this study now opens up a whole new avenue of exploration, and may lead to a possible explanation as to why cell phone use could be linked to increased cancer risk.

Certainly, an increase in brain glucose metabolism can happen during normal brain function, but the question is, can frequently repeated, artificial stimulation of brain glucose metabolism, have serious detrimental effects?

Well, we know that an unnatural increase in brain glucose metabolism can increase free radical production in the brain, which is damaging to healthy cells. In addition, glucose elevation can cause an inflammatory response, which is associated with numerous health problems, including cancer. And, high glucose is clearly linked to insulin resistance, which is in turn linked to Alzheimer's disease, diabetes, and cancer. So, this study may explain how cell phone use can increase cancer risk, and lead to other health problems. (1)

CELL PHONES FOR KIDS

When it comes to cell phone use (as with many modern dangers), we need to take care of our own well being by being proactive. Educate yourself on the potential dangers and find out what you can do to protect yourself, and your loved ones. And, for God's sake, don't give your children cell phones. In ten years we are going to be inundated with a plague of brain tumors amongst our young adults—then who is going to look after all of us baby boomers with Alzheimer's?

Decades ago, European studies linked constant exposure to high EMFs to increased cancer rates, especially in children. If there is anywhere that we should err on the side of caution it is obviously with children, and the failure of the Canadian Health Protection Branch to do so is unconscionable.

In the overview of studies published in Pathophysiology (mentioned at the beginning of this chapter), the study from Sweden found there is a 5 times greater risk of malignant brain tumors in those who begin using cell phones before the age of 20, versus a 1.4% increase in risk for older users.

In Russia, the National Committee on Non Ionizing Radiation Protection advises against the use of cell phones by those 18 years and younger. They warn of the following health risks to children; memory problems, attention deficit, sleep disorders, reduced learning and cognitive abilities, increased irritability and stress, and epilepsy triggers.

Because a child's brain is smaller, and the skull bones thinner, the distance to the antenna is closer to their brain than that of an adult. Therefore, the child's brain absorbs much more electromagnetic radiation than the adult brain does. Unfortunately, safety studies are based on analyzing adult responses, even though children and teenagers will spend as much, or more, time on the phone than most adults. Finally, studies have shown that when developing brains (of rats at least) are exposed to constantly high EMRs, the proper development of the brain is impeded.

And now, with the advent of the smart phone, there is another danger to young people, and this one has nothing to do with the electromagnetic radiation. According to Dr. David Allamby, founder of Focus Clinics (laser eye surgery), the rates of myopia (short sightedness) among young people have increased about 35% since the launch of smart phones (in 1997). He believes the problem could increase by another 50% in the next 10 years. (www.dailymail.co.uk/health/article-2394611)

Should you think this unlikely, consider that, according to the Lancet medical journal, up to 90% of young adults in major East Asian countries, including China, Taiwan, Japan, Singapore and South Korea, are nearsighted—yet 60 years ago, only 10 to 20 percent of the Chinese population was near-sighted.

POSSIBLE CARCINOGEN

After reviewing hundreds of scientific papers on the subject, the World Health Organization's International Agency for Research on Cancer classified electromagnetic radiation fields as a "possible human carcinogen". They came to this conclusion based on a demonstrated increased risk for glioma—a malignant type of brain cancer associated with cell phone use.

"Given the potential consequences for public health of this classification and findings," said IARC director Christopher Wild, "it is important that additional research be conducted into the long-term, heavy use of mobile phones. Pending the availability of such information, it is important to take pragmatic measures to reduce exposure such as hands-free devices or texting."

Critics were quick to point out two things about this announcement. First is, the "possibly carcinogenic" category is used when there is inadequate evidence of cancer-causing effects in humans, but there is sufficient evidence in animals. Second, the human studies used were based on people who already had cancer—people who were expected to remember how often they had used their cell phones, for over more than a decade before they got cancer. And, since their cell phones were (of course) older-style devices, these critics also implied that cell phones are safer now than they were back then.

However, while the cell phones in question may have been older devices, companies have not been required to upgrade their devices to any newer standards (since standards have not changed since then). Also, given that internet access through cell phones is now commonplace, newer phones actually emit much stronger fields than the older ones did.

The response of the British Columbia Cancer Agency to this new classification—rather than erring on the side of caution— was to remind us that public health decisions are not based on the classification of "possible carcinogen". Their argument being, the actual definition means that evidence is limited, and other explanations for the results are possible. At the same time, Bernard Lord, president and CEO of the Canadian Wireless Telecommunications Association, responded that the panel "did not state that there was a direct link to cancer". (And to be fair, the WHO has also applied the definition of "possibly carcinogenic" to substances such as pickled vegetables, and coffee.)

FERTILITY

Many men carry their active cell phone around in pants pockets. Those men who use a Bluetooth device or headset, also carry the phone in a pants pocket, or attached to a holster at the waist. This location of the phone exposes their reproductive organs to cell phone radiation, and some studies have found lower than normal sperm count, and/or poorer sperm quality, in men who carry their phones this way.

French researchers recently revealed that sperm count among the average 35-year-old man has dropped from 73.6 million per milliliter in 1989, to 49.9 million per milliliter in 2005. It is unlikely to be a coincidence that this sudden drop in sperm concentration has occurred following the advent of regular cell phone use—and the evidence bears this out. Studies show exposure to cell phone radiation near the sex organs may lead to decreases in sperm count, sperm motility and vitality, as well as increases in signs of sperm damage, including oxidative stress, DNA damage, and changes in sperm morphology (the size and shape of sperm).

One study found men who carried a phone in a hip pocket, or on the belt, had 11% fewer mobile sperm than men who kept a phone elsewhere on the body. In another study, men who carried their cell phone on the belt, and used it intensively during a five-day test period, had a 19% drop in sperm motility from their previous levels. (2)

Even more shocking, at least 10 studies have revealed simply using a cell phone regularly was enough to reduce fertility, regardless of where one carried it. In fact, one study found men who talked on the phone for more than an hour a day, had 17% fewer highly motile sperm than men who talked for less than 15 minutes daily. This study concluded, "The prolonged use of cell phones may have negative effects on the sperm motility characteristics". (3)

In another (Polish) study, done in 2007, the conclusion was this; "It was also confirmed that a decrease in the percentage of sperm cells in vital progressing motility in the semen is correlated with the frequency of using mobile phones." (4)

In yet another study, sperm parameters were examined in 361 men, undergoing infertility evaluation (2004-2005). Researchers discovered patients who used cell phones more than 4 hours a day had a 42% lower sperm count, and 33% lower sperm motility, than non-users. (5) I have to admit, I find those statistics to be alarming, and something more people should be aware of.

I could find no published studies examining the effect of cell phone radiation on reproductive health in women. Such studies are much more difficult to carry out, since they often require invasive techniques. However, several recent articles have suggested cell phone radiation might be harmful to the developing fetus. For example, a 2009 study done in Turkey, found that after pregnant rats were exposed to cell phone radiation for 15 minutes twice a day, during the entire gestation period, their female pups had fewer ovarian follicles (a sign of reduced fertility). (6)

We also need to consider, if these fields are clearly damaging fertility, then they also have to be a danger to the delicate tissues of the sex organs (ovaries, testes, uterus, and prostate). As if brain tumors were not enough, there may be a host of other potential cancers on the horizon.

OFFSPRING

Now, if these microwaves can damage sperm, and reduce fertility, we have to wonder as well what kind of damage may occur to offspring conceived with such damaged DNA—and some studies do indeed confirm this concern.

A 2012 study, done at Yale University School of Medicine, found that mice exposed to cell phone radiation during gestation were hyperactive, and had impaired memory. (7) There have been similar findings in two human studies: UCLA researchers reported that cell phone exposure during pregnancy, and after birth, was associated with behavioral problems in young children. (8)

As we watch the rise in rates of autism, attention deficit disorder, and hyperactivity, among children and young people, perhaps we should consider restricting their exposure to electrosmog before we start medicating them. As well, perhaps we should start educating parents-to-be about protecting their sperm, eggs, and fetuses, from these prevalent fields.

There is one solution for those who cannot do without their cell phone, and still wish to be fertile, or at least want to prevent behavioral problems in their offspring: Anti-EMF underwear. A company that originally made a belly covering for pregnant women, now also offers specially made boxer briefs for men.

"RadiaShield's" boxer-briefs reduce radiation exposure to male reproductive organs from the front and the back. "The specialized fabric used in the underwear is a highly conductive silver textile (silver woven into cloth), with similar shielding properties to a 1/4-inch thick sheet of aluminum. FCC-certified independent laboratory testing found that RadiaShield boxer-briefs protects male sperm with 99.9 percent effectiveness." (About $50 US: www.bellyarmor.com)

MINIMIZING DAMAGE FROM CELL PHONES

How much of the electromagnetic radiation emitted by cell phones will penetrate your body is dependent on three variables: how close the phone is to your head during calls, the amount of phone calls you make during a day, and how long the calls last. So minimizing use is your first defense.

At home, or where circumstances allow, I suggest using a speakerphone, since the farther you can keep the phone away from your head, the safer it is. Another option at home, or work, is using SKYPE on your computer, set on speaker mode.

Try to use your cell phone mostly in areas that have good reception, since the weaker the reception, the more power the phone uses to transmit. The more power the phone uses the more radiation it emits, and the deeper those waves penetrate into your body.

Avoid carrying the phone on your body, as that adds to your total exposure. Ideally, put it in your purse, backpack, or carrying bag. One woman I know was carrying her cell phone in a holster around her waist, until she started getting unexplained ovarian pain. She then moved it to an ankle holster, and the pains soon ceased.

Keep your cell phone off whenever you can. As long as a cell phone is on, it emits radiation, even when you are not actively using it. One option is to use "Airplane Mode", which will shut off all the transmitting and receiving functions of your phone.

Contrary to popular belief, Bluetooth devices and headsets do not protect the brain from EMR. When using wired headsets make sure that the product is "shielded" (most units are not), otherwise the wire used to transmit the signal to your ear will act as an antenna, transmitting radiation directly to your brain.

The safest kind of headset to use is one with a combination of shielded wire and air-tube. These transmit the signal to your ear as an actual sound wave, and although there are wires involve (shielded in order to protect the rest of the body), no wire goes directly to your head. Hold the actual phone away from your body while using the headset.

Finally, use texting as an option whenever possible.

K. W. PETERS

CORDLESS PHONES

Perhaps you use a cordless phone—during its advent, considered a big step up from being tethered to the old-fashioned landline. If you are one of these non-cell phone users, don't get smug just yet.

When the cordless phone launched in the 1980's, they quickly became ubiquitous. Now we know that cordless phones emit the same type of pulsed microwave radiation as cell phones, and, in most cases, cordless phones are actually more dangerous.

Initially, cordless phones were relatively low power, low-frequency analog devices. Soon however, more "advanced" models became the norm—cordless phones with higher power, and higher frequency pulsed radiation. These types of new cordless phones are based on Digital European Cordless Telephone (DECT) technology, in which both the handset, and the base of the phone, emit pulsed microwave radiation.

Just to re-emphasize, modern cordless phones emit radiation from both the base and the handset, even when not in use. This means, if you are using a DECT cordless phone near the base, you are getting a double dose of microwave radiation.

It wasn't until researchers started to examine the dangers of cell phones (and their potential risk of stimulating brain cancer), that it was realized cordless phones carried the same frequencies as cell phones—and therefore the same risk. This was confirmed by European research, which established that cordless phones raise the risk of developing cancer.

Researchers evaluated phone usage amongst patients with malignant brain tumors, comparing their use of cell phones and DECT cordless phones. What they discovered was cancer risk increased via the use of both types of phones, and worsened by combining the two. (9)

REDUCING THE DANGER OF CORDLESS PHONES

The first and simplest solution is to get rid of your cordless phone, and go back to using a corded phone. The next best solution is to search on-line for a Non DECT cordless phone. Since this concern has already been an issue in Europe for some time now, there are many Non DECT options available. One such model is the Siemens Gigaset ECO Mode Plus, which, if you select the ECO DECT mode when programming the phone, will reduce the transmitting power of the phone's base station by 80%. This model turns off the transmitting power when the phone is in standby mode.

In the meantime, unplug your cordless phone from the wall socket at night, and move the handsets and base at least 6 feet away from areas where you spend the most time. (Remember electromagnetic radiation also goes through walls.) Even when they are unplugged, the charged handsets still emit EMR, as they are always seeking to connect with the base (until their battery has run down).

Another option is to plug in the cordless phone only when you actually need to use it. If you keep at least one corded, landline phone, it will still function if you disconnect the cordless phones. You can hear if someone is trying to ring you, and you will have an answering machine option as well.

Ensure that you do not have a cordless phone base near your bed. This exposes you to 8 hours of damaging frequencies when your body needs to rest and restore, and like all electromagnetic fields, it can interfere with proper sleep patterns.

As with cell phones, the closer the phone is to your head, and the longer the conversations, the more damaging the exposure—so limit the time you talk, and use a speaker phone setting if possible.

PSYCHOLOGICAL ISSUES

In the previous material, I have been discussing the physiological problems with cell phone technology. There is one other issue I would like to address—one that falls into a whole other category.

Since the dawn of time, our primary method of communication, and social learning, has been face-to-face contact. However, since mobile technology has become available to most of the world, digital mediums have increasingly replaced direct human interactions.

Estimations today indicate children in Western countries, aged 8 to 18, spend over 7 hours a day, seven days a week, using digital devices—not including those they use in school. Teenagers now use cell phones, and smartphones, more than any other form of communication, including face-to-face socializing. Now, while they do tend to use these devices more for texting than talking—which at least reduces the exposure of their brains to these dangerous electromagnetic fields—there is another danger to such forms of communication, one that is psychological and emotional in nature.

Studies have found that, from 1997 to 2003, real playtime among children decreased 20%, while screen activities (TV, videogames, computer use) increased, replacing that time. With the latest mobile technology, the youth of today can interact with screens 24/7 outside of school (and somewhat in school, as well). These days, media exposure begins at a very early age, and soon occupies the majority of the free time of young people. This has raised concerns that lack of true human face-to-face interactions is negatively affecting the development of children, and young people.

When we are young, we learn critical social information while engaging in face-to-face communication—most of it from nonverbal cues. These cues are based on the context of the situation, facial expressions, eye contact, and tone of voice. Other factors are body language, posture, and spatial distance between two or more people.

These nonverbal social cues teach us how to modify our behavior in response to the reactions of others, and, what we learn in this manner teaches us how to function properly in society, school, and jobs. Indeed, those who best understand emotional cues in a social environment, are known to develop stronger interpersonal relationships, and superior social skills. This in turn leads to a more successful life, both personally, and in society—be it social, academic, or work-related.

Dr. Iain McGilchrist, a UK psychiatrist, has discovered children today are less empathetic, and less able to read emotions, than the previous generation. Specifically, because they spend too much time interacting via technology. He also has found many of these children are displaying behaviors that are "borderline autistic". McGilchrist maintains, "Small children are not getting the same individual face-to-face attention as before, and when they are at home with the family, the family is multi-tasking and the child is in front of the TV or an iPad screen, which is quite worrying".

He also points out American research shows a decrease in empathy, and a rise in narcissism, among college students. This research, done in 2010 at the University of Michigan, analyzed 72 studies conducted over a 30-year timeframe. It was determined there was a 40% decline in empathy among college students over this period, with most of the decline occurring after 2000. (10)

This particular danger of technology does not necessarily apply to those adults raised during a time of less excessive technological exposure. It is however, clearly affecting the newer generations, and could have a dramatic impact on the psychological well being of both the citizens, and the society which is to follow.

All hope is not lost, though. In 2014, a psychologist did a study on children attending a device-free outdoor camp. He discovered that, after five days without phones or tablets, these children were significantly better at reading facial expressions, and correctly identifying the emotions of actors in videotaped scenes, than the control group.

Of course, the improvement was not due to just avoiding media technology; more importantly, they conversed with each other, and "conversation is the most human and humanizing thing that we do". (11)

So, it is not too late to unplug the children—though good luck getting teenagers to do so—and while I am not suggesting that we turn into Luddites, perhaps there is a middle ground of restrained use.

Endnotes

1. Volkow ND, et al. 2011. "Effects of cell phone radiofrequency signal exposure on brain glucose metabolism." Journal of the American Medical Association 305.
2. Davoudi M, et al. 2002. "The influence of electromagnetic waves on sperm motility." Journal für Urologie und Urogynäkologie 19: 19-22.
3. Arch Androl. 2005 Sep-Oct; 51(5):385-93; "Is there a relationship between cell phone use and semen quality?" Fejes I, et al.
4. Wdowiak A, et al. 2007. "Evaluation of the effect of using mobile phones on male fertility." Ann Agric Environ Med 14(1): 169-72.
5. Agarwal A, et al. 2008. "Effect of cell phone usage on semen analysis in men attending infertility clinic: an observational study." Fertil Steril 89(1): 124-8.
6. Gul A, et al. 2009. "The effects of microwave emitted by cellular phones on ovarian follicles in rats." Arch Gynecol Obstet 280(5): 729-33
7. Aldad TS, et al. 2012. "Fetal radiofrequency radiation exposure from 800-1900 mhz-rated cellular telephones affects neurodevelopment and behavior in mice." Sci Rep 2: 312.
8. Divan HA, et al. 2008. "Prenatal and postnatal exposure to cell phone use and behavioral problems in children." Epidemiology 19(4): 523-9.
9. Pathophysiology 20 (2013) 85–110; "Use of mobile phones and cordless phones is associated with increased risk for glioma and acoustic neuroma." Lennart Hardell et al.

10. "Changes in Dispositional Empathy in American College Students Over Time: A Meta-Analysis." Sara H. Konrath, et al. Pers Soc Psychol Rev 2011 15.

11. Computers in Human Behavior; Volume 39; October 2014, Pages 387–392; "Five days at outdoor education camp without screens improves preteen skills with nonverbal emotion cues." Yalda T. Uhls, et al.

NEUROTRANSMITTERS AND STRESS HORMONES

There are two main areas of the body where damage caused by electrosmog first manifests. One involves the production of neurotransmitters (which are responsible for our moods, as well as certain physiological responses). The other is in the production of stress hormones by our adrenal glands. There, constantly elevated levels of cortisol—our primary stress hormone—leads to a range of ailments that begin with anxiety, and can end up as chronic fatigue. Fortunately, there are nutritional supplements we can take to boost our neurotransmitter production back to healthful levels, and other supplements that can help us cope with excessive cortisol.

In 2011, researchers reported on changes in neurotransmitter and hormonal levels in a group of volunteers who had lived near a new cell tower (erected in Rimbach, Austria), for about one and a half years. The hormones examined were epinephrine and norepinephrine, and the neurotransmitters tracked were dopamine and phenylethylamine (PEA).

All had been affected by exposure to the cell tower. Epinephrine and norepinephrine levels increased significantly during the first six months, while dopamine and PEA levels decreased dramatically. (1)

By the end of the study, the levels of these compounds had not been restored to their original levels, and incidences of allergies, headaches, dizziness, and problems with sleep and concentration, were seen more frequently in the subjects. The authors of this study suggested cell tower radiation generated a chronic stress response in the residents—explaining the great variety of illnesses, and increased death rates, reported in people who live near cell towers.

NEUROTRANSMITTERS

Neurotransmitters are chemical messengers that send signals from one nerve cell to another, and, when it comes to our moods, a proper balance of them is required for healthy functioning. There are two basic classes of neurotransmitters: excitory and inhibitory. The excitory ones—acetylcholine, dopamine and PEA—give us our "get up and go", and "joie de vivre". They make us happy, reward us for learning and falling in love, and motivate us to get up in the morning. The inhibitory ones—serotonin and GABA—allow us to relax, feel calm, cope with stress, and sleep.

Neurotransmitter production can be faulty due to many aspects of modern living, including personal trauma, poor nutrition, bad genes, drug addiction, physical injuries, and various disease states. The prevalence of anti-anxiety and anti-depression medications indicates just how widespread neurotransmitter malfunctions are. Since we can now add electrosmog to the list of things that impede proper neurotransmitter production, the number of people seeking medication for anxiety and/or depression will likely not be dropping anytime soon.

In the aforementioned study, levels of the neurotransmitter dopamine dropped significantly during the first year, while the PEA levels remained unchanged for the first 6 months, and then plummeted over the course of the subsequent year. Since adequate amounts of dopamine and PEA are required for us to feel happy and good about life, it is easy to see how electrosmog can cause depression by reducing these neurotransmitters.

DOPAMINE

The brain has several distinct dopamine systems, one of which plays a major role in reward-motivated behavior. Most types of reward increase the level of dopamine in the brain, including learning new things (making connections in the brain), and falling in love. A wide range of addictive drugs also increase dopamine neuronal activity—from sugar and coffee, to cocaine and heroin. Other brain dopamine systems are involved in motor control, and controlling the release of other important hormones.

Because of this involvement in motor control, a loss of dopamine-secreting neurons, or dopamine receptors, has been identified as a cause of Parkinson's disease—characterized by tremors, and loss of balance and motor control. Other diseases of the nervous system have also been associated with dysfunctions of the dopamine system.

Recent research shows the vitamin D receptor is most strongly expressed in those areas of the brain that are richest in dopamine. This may explain why vitamin D has proven helpful in slowing the progression of Parkinson's disease, as well as other neurological conditions. Therefore, we should consider vitamin D an important part of our arsenal in the fight against electromagnetic pollution.

It should be mentioned that dopamine is also required for the production of melanin in the body. Melanin gives skin its pigment, so observing sections of your skin losing pigment, or being diagnosed with full-blown vitiligo—although there are other causes of vitiligo as well—can be indicative of low dopamine levels.

Fortunately, there are a number of supplements which can naturally elevate dopamine levels. Following are some dopamine precursors.

- Avena Sativa: flowering green oat extract—Avenaforce from Vogel is one of the best—take as directed.

- L-Tyrosine: 500-1000 mg, 1 to 3 times daily, on an empty stomach.

- Phosphatidylserine: 100 mg, 1 to 3 times daily, with food.

- Mucuna Puriens: an Ayurvedic herb available as powder, or an extract in capsules; take as directed.

- SAMe: S-Adenosyl methionine—so strong it is prescribed as an anti-depressant in Europe—start with a low dose, 200 mg, one to three times daily, as it can be agitating for some people, although high doses are recommended for arthritis, and liver malfunction.

PHENYLETHYLAMINE

PEA is another neurotransmitter found in the central nervous system, biosynthesized in the body from the amino acid L-phenylalanine. Abnormally low concentrations of PEA are found in those with attention deficit hyperactivity disorder, and abnormally high concentrations have been linked to schizophrenia. PEA is concentrated in the limbic system (the brain's emotional center), and increases motivation, physical drive, feelings, and social activity. It also has the ability to facilitate the release of noradrenalin, and dopamine.

PEA has been described as the "love drug", because it mimics the brain chemistry of a person in love. This is the reason why chocolate, which contains an appreciable amount of PEA, is said to be an aphrodisiac.

To elevate PEA, one can take the amino acid L-phenylalanine (500-1000 mg, 1 to 3 times daily, on an empty stomach), and/or eat copious amounts of chocolate (ideally organic, dark chocolate, with minimal sugar). There is now also a supplemental form of phenylethylamine hydrochloride on the market, taken at a dosage of 300 mg, one to three times daily. (I have yet to see it for sale in Canadian vitamin stores, but it can be purchased online.) However, a friend of mine had a very unpleasant experience when taking pure PEA, so it may be safer to stick with the precursor, L-phenylalanine.

STRESS HORMONES

As the Austrian cell tower study indicated, not only do these electromagnetic fields lower positive neurotransmitters, but they also elevate levels of the stress hormones—epinephrine and norepinephrine. Epinephrine and norepinephrine, also known as adrenaline and noradrenaline, are secreted by the adrenal glands. Adrenaline is known as the "fight or flight" hormone because it is released at times of high stress, and its stimulatory effects prepare an animal for one, or the other, of those actions.

While the actions of epinephrine and norepinephrine are generally similar, they differ from each other in certain biological effects. However, both are considered stress hormones. Both hormones increase the rate and force of contraction of the heart, increasing output of blood from the heart, and raising blood pressure. Epinephrine also stimulates the conversion of glycogen to glucose in the liver, which results in increased blood sugar levels, explaining, in part, why increased risk of diabetes is often associated with exposure to electromagnetic pollution.

If that is not bad enough, we now know the other major stress hormone, cortisol, is also elevated by constant exposure to high intensity fields of electromagnetic radiation.

CORTISOL

The negative health effects of chronic cortisol stimulation are well known in the medical profession, though the link between EMR exposure and excess cortisol production has yet to be acknowledged by conventional medicine (even though animal studies clearly show this effect).

Cortisol is also released by the adrenal glands, and it serves as an effective part of a short-term solution to danger, by helping adrenaline mobilize resources for the fight or flight response. However, when cortisol is continuously secreted, it wreaks havoc on the body. High cortisol is linked to a variety of ailments including, anxiety, autoimmune disorders, stress-induced hypertension, various inflammatory conditions, insomnia (especially indicated when wakefulness occurs at 3 or 4 am), the breakdown of connective tissue, poor memory, and the accumulation of abdominal fat. Abdominal fat—with its link to diabetes, and its constant proliferation of estrogen-like compounds—is easily the most dangerous kind of adipose tissue.

Modern studies are beginning to reveal that electromagnetic fields cause some of their damage by elevating cortisol levels, as this one study concluded: "These results indicate that 900 MHz EMF emitted by cellular telephones in long term exposure increased serum cortisol and T4 levels and decreased T3 level in Syrian Hamster, and it can destroy endocrine system generally." (2) The T3 and T4 referenced here are thyroid hormones, suggesting the thyroid is also negatively affected by EMFs.

In another, older study, involving cows, the animals exposed to EMFs showed an increase in blood pressure, heart rate, and cortisol levels, as well as a reduction in oxytocin (a feel-good hormone that encourages bonding). This response did not occur in the control animals not exposed to electromagnetic fields. (3) (Note the previous two studies examined EMR effects on stress hormones, while this one examined EMFs, as does the following rat study. The bottom line is all forms of electromagnetic pollution negatively affect the stress hormones.)

ADRENAL FATIGUE

This increased cortisol level in cows, caused by short-term EMF exposure, concurs with results observed in rats. However, in this case, the rats were subjected to these fields for periods of up to two years (and long-term exposure has a very different effect on cortisol).

In this rat study, the rats all began with equal levels of blood cortisol; shortly after the experiment began, rats exposed to the electromagnetic field had their cortisol levels rise. However, by the time the experiment ended, cortisol levels in the exposed rats were actually much lower than those of the controls. This pattern is commonly observed in those constantly exposed to high levels of stress; the adrenal glands cannot maintain production of excessive amounts of cortisol, and they eventually crash, resulting in adrenocortical fatigue. (4)

By the time the adrenal glands are so depleted they cannot produce sufficient amounts of cortisol for day-to-day functioning, we begin to see symptoms such as depression, fatigue, muscle weakness, extremely low blood pressure, weight loss, and changes in mood and personality. This can progress to kidney failure, severe abdominal pains, chronic fatigue syndrome, and Addison's disease.

Another clue one has reached adrenal burnout is edema. When the body is lacking in cortisol, it is unable to produce adequate amounts of a hormone (aldosterone) required to clear water from the body.

When produced at optimal levels, cortisol is necessary for suppressing inflammatory processes in the body. However, when adrenal function is low, cortisol levels may not be adequate to keep these inflammatory processes in check; so, for example, arthritis pain may flare up.

Corticosteroids (synthetic cortisol) are often prescribed for inflammatory conditions, such as arthritis and psoriasis. While this can be helpful in the short term, these drugs suppress natural cortisol production, and eventually seriously impair adrenal, and immune, functions.

It is impossible to maintain optimal adrenal function while taking strong corticosteroids, and it can take a long time for adrenal function to recover, after being on these drugs for an extended period. If you have been on corticosteroids for any significant length of time, you should work with an alternative health practitioner to come off the drug, find natural alternatives to address the inflammatory condition, and rebuild your adrenal glands.

I will make a final, unsettling point here: both the cows and the rats, in their respective studies, were subjected to EMF fields lower than levels currently approved by the FCC, and Congressional Telecommunications Act of 1996, as acceptable for human exposure.

COLLAGEN

Excess cortisol in the body also inhibits collagen synthesis, and reduced collagen production leads to another variety of health issues. Collagen is the "glue" that holds us together, and is an important component of cartilage, connective tissue, the intestinal tract, blood vessels, and skin.

Symptoms of low collagen include thinning of the skin, thinning of the walls of capillaries (which can lead to bleeding within the skin and a tendency toward unexplained bleeding), gastrointestinal disorders, ulcers, acid reflux, and joint and/or muscle pain.

Collagen synthesis is supported by regularly ingesting either bone broth, or a collagen supplement (marine, bovine, or porcine-derived). Even old-fashioned gelatin (which is cooked collagen) can be helpful for maintaining healthy collagen levels. Nutrients that help build and maintain collagen include vitamins C and E, the mineral silica, and the amino acids L-proline and L-lysine.

Another potential symptom of excess cortisol is osteoporosis. Cortisol inhibits bone formation by reducing Type 1 collagen formation (important for bone strength and flexibility), and by reducing the production of osteoblasts (cells which synthesize new bone tissue). As well, cortisol disrupts the uptake of vitamin D, thereby decreasing absorption of calcium from the intestines, resulting in an overall reduction in bone mass.

DIABETES

We are not finished with cortisol yet. Cortisol is also involved in producing glucose from protein. While this primarily involves storing glucose as glycogen in the liver (aka carb-loading), which is a good thing, excess cortisol will eventually increase blood glucose levels, which is not a good thing.

Increased blood glucose levels occur because cortisol is antagonistic to the actions of insulin on glucose metabolism, inhibiting insulin-stimulated glucose uptake into muscle and fat tissue, and reversing the insulin suppression of glucose production in the liver.

In other words, chronically high cortisol levels are directly linked to increasing the risk of developing diabetes. Indeed, an Australian study showed the incidence of Type II diabetes was higher among people living near power transmission lines, and was positively correlated to daily exposure rates (amount of time spent under the influence of the EMFs). (5)

CONTROLLING CORTISOL

Keeping cortisol under control is done by using a combination of stress-reduction methods (such as breathing control techniques, meditation, yoga, or Tai Chi), and taking supplements that support adrenal function. Most of the herbs used for adrenal support are considered adaptogenic, meaning they are substances that help organisms deal with stress.

This subject is covered in Volume One of Health Secrets, but here is a brief list of the best adaptogens to look for: ashwaganda, holy basil, licorice root, rhodiola, panax ginseng, Siberian ginseng, schisandra, and/or suma. These substances can be taken individually, or in a combination found in one of the many adrenal support formulas on the market (including one I designed for NutriStart Vitamin Company, called Adrenal Start).

Aside from the herbal support provided by adaptogens, when the adrenals are under extreme stress, we need to provide them with extra vitamin C (500–1000 mg, 3 times daily), and vitamin B5 (Pantothenic Acid–250 mg, 3 times daily).

Some formulas will also use animal adrenal extracts (from cows or pigs) to treat severe conditions, especially when in the final stages of adrenal exhaustion. Adrenal extracts contain small amounts of naturally occurring adrenaline, which can serve to "prime the pump", and jumpstart the adrenal glands into producing natural cortisol again.

PHOSPHATIDYLSERINE

Phosphatidylserine (PS) is another excellent supplement that keeps cortisol in check, and has the bonus function of repairing damaged brain cells. PS is so effective at repairing brain damage it is often prescribed for those suffering side effects from physical trauma to the head.

PS is a phospholipid, which is a type of fat critical for cell membrane function. Phospholipids help to maintain cell membrane structure, and move nutrients into and out of the cells. As a superior phospholipid, PS can increase the efficiency of cell membranes, revitalize membrane function, and protect cell membranes from damage.

While PS is needed for maintenance of cell membranes throughout the body, it is found in highest concentrations in the nerve cells of the brain. Thus, it is used to treat symptoms of poor memory, concentration, and cognition, as well as Alzheimer's disease, dementia, and mood disorders. PS works on mood disorders by elevating levels of brain neurotransmitters (not just dopamine, but also acetylcholine, norepinephrine, and serotonin), and reducing damage to nerve cells.

PS is perhaps my favorite supplement for dealing with damage caused by electromagnetic pollution because it singlehandedly compensates for three of the worst things electrosmog does to us. PS lowers cortisol, raises dopamine, and repairs and protects cell membranes (as you may recall, ruptured cell walls are a significant trauma EMFs can cause). The therapeutic dose for PS is 100 mg, three times daily, with food.

Endnotes

1. Buchner K, Eger H (2011); "Changes of Clinically Important Neurotransmitters under the Influence of Modulated RF Fields - A Long-term Study under Real-life Conditions." Umwelt-Medizin-in-Gesellschaft 24(1): 44-57.
2. Endocrine Abstracts (2009) 20 P73; "Effects of 900 MHz electromagnetic fields emitted from cellular phone on T3, T4 and cortisol hormones of Syrian Hamsters (Mesocricetus auratus)"; Habib Aghdam Shahryar & Alireza Lotfi.
3. Gorewit, R.C., et al. "Effects of electrical current on milk production and animal health." American Society of Agricultural Engineers Annual International Meeting Technical Paper No. 84:3502–3520. ASAE, St. Joseph, MI; 1984.
4. Becker, Robert O. 1990. "Cross Currents, The Perils of Electropollution– the Promise of Electromedicine.: Jeromy P. Tarcher/Perigee Books, The Putnam Publishers, New York, NY.
5. Beale, Ivan L., et al. 2001. "Association of health problems with 50 hz magnetic fields in human adults living near power transmission lines." J. Australian College of Nutritional & Environmental Medicine 20(2): 9-12 and 15-30.

PROTECTION FROM ELECTROMAGNETIC POLLUTION

Now that many people are aware of the ill effects of electromagnetic pollution, a whole new industry has arisen to help us cope with these damaging fields—though the solutions offered range from the scientifically valid, to the dubious, and esoteric. If you have no tolerance for the dubious and esoteric, bear with me: the more scientifically valid technologies will follow soon.

Q-LINK AND EARTHCALM

I am fortunate in that I am not overly sensitive to electrosmog, nonetheless I do feel the need to use some form of protection (an ounce of prevention…). Many professionals (including Ken Wilber, some musicians, and star athletes) endorse the Q-link (www.qlink-products.com), which comes as a pendent, or bracelet, and claims to protect the body against all forms of electrosmog.

To quote from Q-link, "At the heart of all Q-Link® products is Sympathetic Resonance Technology. SRT™ is an array of proprietarily identified frequencies that support and enhance the efficiency and performance of various organic and inorganic systems".

I personally chose to use "Earthcalm" products—both a device for the house, and a pendant for my body. I decided on this product based on testimonials from people who are hypersensitive to electromagnetic pollution. As well, Earthcalm has been in business for 25 years, suggesting that maybe they are onto something. EarthCalm products use what they call "Scalar Resonance Technology", based on "proprietary geometric circuits, which mirror the structure of the earth's electromagnetic field, and amplify your resonance with the earth". (www.earthcalm.com)

Another, newer, player in the field of protective pendants is Biogetica, a company specializing in Ayurvedic medicine. They define their Resonam pendants as "advanced bio feedback devices, which harmonize hertzian and non hertzian frequencies in the bio energy field, and protect one from electromagnetic and high frequency radiations". (www.biogetica.com)

Besides pendants, and plug-in devices (for wall outlets, or USB ports), another version of esoteric technology are small disks that are attached to the computer, cell phone, or other electronic devices. These disks claim to neutralize the ill effects of electromagnetic fields. (Examples include, The Neutralizer, from Aulterra, at www.aulterra.com, and Fusion Excel Shields, found at www.fusionexcel.ca.)

PSEUDOSCIENCE?

Now, these products would fall under the category I referred to as esoteric—meaning there is no current scientific acceptance of how they work. I must admit, the explanations of how these products work sounds dubious, from a scientific perspective. This is the problem with many of these devices designed to counteract electrosmog: the science on them is on the fringe, to say the least.

These types of devices are generally "proven" through kinesiology (muscle-testing), or thermal imaging of the brain (which shows less heating up of brain material when the devices are used). Or, effectiveness is demonstrated through live blood cell analysis, which shows less platelet clumping when the devices are used, compared to when blood cells are exposed to electromagnetic pollution without the device. These are somewhat valid testing techniques, though, it could be claimed responses are due to the placebo effect.

You cannot measure the protective effect of such devices with a gauss meter, since if they stopped the actual electromagnetic waves (such as with a Faraday cage), your wireless connection, or cell phone, would no longer work. What most of these devices claim to do is to create counter (or scalar) waves, to neutralize the ill effects of those frequencies not healthy to living organisms.

The definition of a scalar wave is one generated whenever one wave is matched in frequency, and amplitude, by another wave—such that they cancel each other out. However, according to www.rationalwiki.org (a site that debunks pseudoscience), "A scalar wave is a purported type of electromagnetic wave that works outside physics as we know it...the term "scalar wave" is used exclusively by cranks and peddlers of woo".

However, the fact is, science does not embrace new concepts very well. It has a tendency to be an entrenched, myopic system that thinks too highly of itself, and has no time for concepts that do not fall into its predetermined scientific categories. Many advances in knowledge come from renegades, outside the field of accepted science, in part, because those people do not have the same blinders on.

For example, acupuncture was rejected by science for decades, then, in the 70s, we developed machinery sensitive enough to detect the little energy vortexes located at the acupuncture points. Yet, those points were mapped out thousands of years ago, by humans without such machines. As well, homeopathy to this day is considered quackery by most scientists, but has over a hundred years of effective use in alternative medicine.

So, I suggest trying to keep an open mind on the subject, since many of these products do in fact work for a lot of people, and it seems unlikely the placebo effect can work on electromagnetic sensitivity.

Science may mock homeopathy, and scalar waves, but when

we consider that, in 2013, the Journal of the American Medical Association reported that SSRI antidepressants are little better than placebo for most cases of depression (after reviewing 30 years of data), maybe their recommendations shouldn't be trusted either.

A MORE SCIENTIFIC APPROACH

The original anti-EMF products, which could be measured with current technology—and be proven effective, scientifically—came out of Europe, as electromagnetic pollution was an issue there, long before North America woke up to it. Now, such products are also available in North America, found in specialty stores, and commonly available on-line (simply search for "emf protection").

These initial forms of protection against electrosmog are in the form of copper-based paints and wallpaper, and clothing and fabrics containing metal mesh (fine screening). Such forms of protection are based on the principles of a Faraday Cage. A Faraday Cage is a (grounded) copper mesh box (of varying sizes) designed to test sensitive electronic equipment: the mesh cage breaks up electromagnetic waves, so they cannot affect the device being calibrated, or tested.

Metal mesh fabrics are used to make protective clothing, such as a baseball-style cap, with an earflap that unfolds to cover the ear when you use a cell phone. As well, there are scarves available that can be wrapped around the head, when using a cell phone; other clothing covers the top of the body—where most of the sensitive organs are—and there are even underwear to protect fertility.

Bed coverings, and clothing articles, are made with copper, silver, or aluminum mesh, woven into the fabric. Or, for cheaper, though less effective, products, Mylar is used (easily obtained by purchasing emergency blankets), and, even simple aluminum mesh screening, from the hardware store, is a fairly effective blocker.

From our current scientific model, these metal-based mesh products are probably the most sound. For example, if you wrap your cell phone in Mylar it won't receive a signal, or, if you put aluminum screening between your testing meter and a cordless phone, or smart meter, you can see it will block the signal.

One of the best sources for Electromagnetic Field Shielding products—including EMF shielding paints, plastics, fabrics & foils, netting for the bed, and personal shielding for computers, cell phones, and a variety of clothing—is www.lessemf.com. Another good company is www.slt.

Now, most of these forms of shielding will be most effective when they are grounded (though, of course, this is not possible with hats, and clothing). Grounding wires, that run from the Mylar, or mesh fabric, to the grounding outlet in the wall, or to a metal rod stuck into the ground outside, can be found on sites that sell anti-EMF products (including the ones mentioned above).

A MIX OF ESOTERIC AND SCIENTIFIC

One interesting device, developed to help neutralize harmful electromagnetic pollution, is the "Total Shield". This unit is designed to cover an area of about 20,000 square feet, and claims to protect a home, or work, environment against harmful geopathic disturbances, EMFs, EMR, and RFs.

Total Shield is comprised of two separate electronic generators. One generator is a detector device that identifies the frequencies of the electromagnetic disturbances, and broadcasts them back out through a Tesla coil, which cancels out the disturbance. Since this approach is essentially functioning based on the scalar wave theory, this component would qualify as esoteric, or pseudoscience—depending on your belief system.

On the other hand, the other generator is a 7.83 frequency generator, which duplicates the Schumann resonance—the resonant frequency of the Earth's magnetic field—and the Schumann resonance is based on a measurable, scientifically sound principle.

Exposure to the Schumann frequency is necessary for good health, and in fact, NASA created machines to simulate these waves in space capsules, because humans cannot survive without them. Unfortunately, Schumann waves are blocked by modern building materials such as concrete, which presents a problem in urban areas, and especially in high rise apartments, where the higher up you are, the more you are removed from exposure to this healthy frequency.

My frequently mentioned friend (hypersensitive to electromagnetic pollution), has found the Total Shield to be a highly effective product, improving her health demonstrably. The Total Shield retails for about $400 US (for the basic model) and is available from www. brimhall.com.

REDUCING EXPOSURE

For our health to be negatively impacted by electromagnetic pollution, we have to be exposed to it for long periods. Of course now, since the advent of cell phone towers, smart meters, and Wi-Fi, we are all exposed to these fields consistently, and they are almost impossible to escape. But, we can try to minimize our exposure wherever possible, and knowing the worst offenders is a good place to begin.

The worst offenders for standard electronic EMFs are, computers, and electronic cash registers (when you work behind them for extended periods), laptops (when you hold them on your lap), electric blankets, and electric clock radios (except when battery operated).

One's head should be at least 3 to 4 feet away from a clock radio (the type that is plugged into the wall), since they put out a 4-foot radius of EMFs. If you are within this field, you will be suppressing your melatonin levels at the very time you are trying to sleep.

Though landline phones do not put out microwaves (like cell phones), I have found some of these phones to produce higher EMF levels than cell phones (and cordless phones are even worse than landlines), when using them. If your ear starts to burn after 20 minutes, or so, on the phone, or you start to develop a headache, then it is clearly producing high levels of damaging frequencies.

Power lines (electrical transmission lines) are one of the worst sources of EMFs, and it is quite dangerous to live near them. Some power lines carry such high voltages that they emit high levels of EMFs for up to 1/4 mile on either side of the line. Many studies have found links between living near power lines and higher rates of brain and breast cancer, leukemia (especially in children), birth defects and reproductive problems, depression, heart disease, sleeping complaints, and a host of other ailments. If you live under or near power lines, your only real option is to move. (1)

But, you don't have to live under the transmission lines to be exposed to unsafe levels of EMF pollution from hydro lines. I have tested a bedroom that showed constant, dangerously high EMF levels, due to a power transmitter across the street. In this case, the main power line was running from the transformer into the top of the house, just above that bedroom. I then used a gauss meter to find the safest spot in which to locate the bed.

Many years ago, I found that one of my boy's bed was in a high EMF zone, due to the power box in the garage being located directly below his bed. Again, I used the gauss meter to determine a safer place to locate the bed.

WHAT YOU CAN DO TO PROTECT YOURSELF

- Eliminate Wi-Fi in the home, and instead use a hard-wired broadband connection. Same goes for wireless baby monitors, and wireless speakers.

- Do not use CFLs (compact fluorescent light-bulbs). CFLs emit high levels of EMFs as a byproduct of the energy-saving mechanism used to reduce voltage. You can prove this by holding an AM radio close to a lit CFL bulb, and hearing the disruption of the radio signal. Interestingly, AM radio serves as a rough gauss meter, since the radio signal will become contaminated with static when you are in the proximity of high electromagnetic fields. A small AM radio can also be used around the house to roughly detect strong fields. CLFs are also to be avoided because of the danger of mercury contamination, should they break.

- Use only incandescent bulbs at any location where you will be within 6 feet of the light source. LED bulbs are a viable alternative, as they are low voltage, so they only radiate appreciable EMFs for about 12 inches out from source (and they are mercury-free).

- Avoid dimmers, fluorescent, High Intensity Lighting (HID), Metal Halide, arc lamps, or any other lighting besides conventional incandescent bulbs (or LED).

- Wherever possible, replace cell phones, and cordless phones, with a corded landline phone.

- Use scientifically-proven EMR protective devices for the home and body, such as EMR-protective clothing for the body, and shielding paint or wallpaper for the home (resources to follow).

CELL PHONE TOWERS

For too long, my hypersensitive friend lived within a few blocks of a cell phone tower array. There she often felt like she was being literally cooked alive and, had to use a combination of mylar shielding, and aluminum mesh, as well as a few other devices, in order to survive in that environment. Since these towers are putting out microwaves, she was not far off with her sensation of being cooked.

She has high mercury levels, and, in the natural health field, it is acknowledged that people with high levels of heavy metals are much more sensitive to electromagnetic pollution. It is possible the metals literally act like antennas in their blood, amplifying the signals. If you suspect you have high levels of heavy metals in your body, you can find out by getting a hair analysis, or a live blood cell analysis. If this is confirmed, you should follow a heavy metal detoxification protocol.

If you live near a cell phone tower, and you have any serious health problems, you should investigate some protective measures to insulate yourself from the harmful effects of this radiation (resources to follow). If you are not sure, hire a technician, or buy a meter, to check the levels of electromagnetic pollution in your home generally, and your bedroom particularly. (A list of consultants in your area can be found at, www.electricsense.com.)

If test readings show you are in the danger zone, your best solution is simply to move; the situation is not going to change, and the hazards to health only increase over time. In the meantime, you can use the aforementioned anti-EMR paints, or wallpapers, and hang anti-EMR netting over the windows for curtains. If this is too much expense, or work, for you, then focus on the bedroom, so you at least have a sanctuary during the 8, or so, hours you are trying rest and recuperate.

PROTECTION FROM SMART METERS

If you own your own house, in some places it is possible to have the smart meter replaced with an old analog device (often along with paying a monthly fee for this exemption). If you live in an apartment or condo complex, this will not be an option.

The more time you spend close to a smart meter, the more it will affect your health. So, if it is located near your bedroom, living room, or home office, the more imperative it is that you do something to protect yourself.

It is difficult to protect an entire house, so if you must choose one room to protect from smart meter RFs, it should be the bedroom. You can use the RF reflecting carbon-based paints, or copper-based wallpaper, or silver netting. Some people will just use thick aluminum foil, or Mylar, but, in this case, you need to ground it (attach a wire to the foil, and plug this into the ground inlet on a wall socket, or take it outside and attach it to a metal rod sunk into the earth). Shielding and grounding products can be found at www.lessemf. com.

Ideally (given the resources), one would line the entire bedroom with these protective shields, but, at the very least, one should cover the wall that has the smart meter on the other side.

PROTECTING THE BEDROOM

Sleeping in a room with devices emitting EMFs will only worsen health issues that stem from proximity to cell phone towers, wireless signals, and smart meters. This occurs because, aside from the host of ailments and symptoms already discussed, EMF exposure suppresses melatonin production, interrupting sleep cycles. Thus, because of the necessity of sleep and melatonin for good health, electrosmog exposure is most dangerous at night.

- Don't keep a cell phone in the bedroom unless it is switched to "Airplane mode", otherwise it will be emitting and receiving signals while you are trying to sleep.

- Remove any cordless phones from the bedroom, and, if you must have a phone in that room, use a regular corded landline.

- Shut down all computer devices in the bedroom, and all wireless routers in the house, at night.

- Use a battery-powered alarm clock, and do not sleep under an electric blanket. You can use an electric blanket to warm the bed before you get into it, but do not sleep under it, if it is plugged in.

- Ensure that electrical devices like TVs, stereos, air conditioner units, and refrigerators, are at least 6 feet away from where you sleep. That also means at least 6 feet away vertically as well, since electrical frequencies from those devices can pass through floors and walls. Also make sure your fuse box is no closer than 6 feet from your bed (again, also in a vertical sense, that is, above or below the bed as well).

- If you are hypersensitive to electrosmog, and still not sleeping well after following some of the preceding recommendations, or you if are showing other symptoms (anxiety, breathing difficulties, unusual inflammation), you can also consider cutting off the power supply to your bedroom before going to bed. (Have a battery-powered light available.) If you do not know which circuit breaker shuts off power in the bedroom, leave the lights on and switch off the circuits one by one until you find the right one (or possibly two).

- If you are having sleep problems that cannot be naturally resolved, or if your heart races when you try to sleep, create a bed canopy from "shielding" fabric. This is a silver-lined net (like a mosquito net) that filters out 99% of high-frequency EMR.

These shielding fabrics are especially good for dealing with exposure to cell tower radiation, along with other forms of electrosmog, but it is important in this case that the bed be fully enclosed. This requires using a piece of this special fabric that goes under the bed, and meets the fabric that hangs from above—otherwise the omnipresent EMR will come up from underneath.

Two good shielding fabrics are made by Swiss Shield (polyester base), and Naturell (cotton base), both available (along with a variety of other protective products) from www.radmeters.com.

BEWARE THE MATTRESS

According to an article in Scientific American, breast cancer and melanoma (both on the increase) occurs 10% more frequently on the left side of the body, than on the right. In an attempt to explain this, researchers looked to Japan. In Japan there is no correlation between melanoma and breast cancer rates (unlike in the West), and there is no left-side prevalence for either disease. (2)

The difference in cancer rates (and left-side prevalence) between Japan and the Western countries, may be a result of the difference in beds used by the two cultures. A link between bedroom furniture and cancer may seem absurd, but according to research, this is the answer.

This bed-based cancer theory originated from a 2007 study in Sweden (conducted between 1989 and 1993), revealing a strong link between incidences of melanoma, and the number of FM, and TV, transmission towers, in areas where the affected individuals lived.

COIL SPRING ANTENNA

It seems our coil-spring mattresses (and metal bed frames) are in effect functioning as antennas—amplifying broadcast FM/TV radiation—exposing us to amplified electromagnetic radiation while we sleep. (In Japan, most beds are not made of metal; frames are wood, and futons have no metal coils.)

The problem worsens when an electric blanket is used, as electric energy from the blanket transfers into the mattress coils, amplifying its field. It is also likely that mattress coils pick up, and store, other harmful electromagnetic frequencies—including those from cordless phones, cell phone towers, wireless routers, and smart meters.

According to this theory, the solution is to use a cotton futon, or latex mattress—which do not contain metal coils—and choose wood instead of metal, for bed frames and headboards.

To find out if a bed contains a residual electromagnetic charge, one can use a liquid-filled compass. While holding the compass above the bed, see if the needle spins instead of pointing to magnetic north. If so, the bed is holding residual electromagnetism.

Another way to test a bed is to use a meter that measures skin voltage (body voltage meter). If your body voltage levels rise when laying on the bed, you will know the mattress has an adverse charge. A body voltage meter is a very valuable tool for those who are hypersensitive to electromagnetic frequencies. (Body voltage meters are available from www.lessemf.com.)

MOLD

If mold is present in a house, due to structural damage, lack of air circulation, or just dampness from living near the ocean, it will thrive in the presence of EMFs of all types. I have seen this occur in the house of my friend who lived near a bank of cell phone towers; there mold developed far faster than normal—on food, in the fish tank, and on plants.

Mold can severely affect health, seriously compromising one's immune system. And, it can produce even more dangerous compounds, known as mycotoxins. Once these get into the body, they contribute to a wide range of health problems including asthma and lung problems, cancer, cardiovascular disease, impaired kidney and liver function, insomnia, and brain fog.

Dr. Dietrich Klinghardt (a specialist in mercury detox), discusses on his website how it was discovered electromagnetic pollution increases mold growth. A Swiss scientist compared mold cultures grown in a faraday cage (which blocks all EMFs), with mold exposed to the ambient electromagnetic pollution found in his laboratory.

When exposed to electrosmog from computers, lights, and a nearby cell phone tower, the molds increased their production of bio-toxins by over 600 times (compared to mold shielded from these frequencies). Evidently, those toxins were not only in higher quantities, but also more potent and dangerous, than in their original form. (www.klinghardtacademy.com)

This discovery could partially explain the rise of antibiotic-resistant "superbugs" that are a growing problem in modern hospitals— these buildings are loaded with electronic equipment of all types, often including cell phone antennas on the roof.

It may also be one reason why some people are hypersensitive to electromagnetic pollution: if those people have candida fungus, mold, or other microbial infections, in their blood already, such exposure to these fields could amplify and worsen their conditions.

DEALING WITH MOLD

If you suspect mold may be a problem in your household, there are some safety measures you can take. Stay on top of cleaning, especially where mold is most likely to thrive—in damp environments (around showers, sinks, and tubs). Use a vacuum cleaner with a HEPA filter for your carpets, and use a HEPA air filter in your home. It is also helpful to use a dehumidifier to keep the humidity low in rooms prone to mold, such as the basement, and bathrooms.

For optimal effectiveness, choose an air filter that also is an ionizer, and/or buy a "negative ion" generator, since both ionizers, and negative ion machines, will purify the air of low levels of mold, bacteria, and toxins. For buildings with serious mold contamination (for example, in the walls) you will need to contact a mold remediation expert (easily found online).

For information on safely removing mold from your house, and when it might be time to bring in an expert, visit this website, www.blacktoxicmolds.com.

They discuss the low-tech approach of using vinegar or bleach to kill superficial mold, but suggest an even better mold-killer is borax. Borax is one of the strongest mold-killing agents, and unlike bleach, borax does not emit dangerous gases (and is not as bad for the environment as bleach).

Following are the basics of using borax.

- Mix borax with water, at a ratio of one cup of borax to one gallon of hot water, ensuring the borax is fully dissolved into the water. (Borax can irritate the skin so one should wear rubber gloves just to be safe.) This solution can be used in a spray bottle, or you can make a paste of borax and water, and spread it onto moldy areas.

- Apply the borax and water solution to moldy areas, and let sit for a few minutes. Then use a brush, cloth, or paper towels, to wipe the mold away. Rinsing afterward is unnecessary since the lingering borax will help prevent mold from returning.

- Borax can also be added to your washing machine, in order to remove mold and mildew from clothing and fabrics. (1/2 cup fully dissolved in hot water, then added to water in washing machine.)

MOLD IN THE BODY

Fortunately, certain supplements have the ability to kill mold internally, if used regularly. A live blood cell analysis (available through naturopaths) can be used to determine if one is harboring excessive candida, mold, yeast, or microbes.

Even if one just suspects they have mold issues, it is reasonable to start a slow-killing regimen. However, killing mold and bad bacteria too fast can cause die-off symptoms, leading one to feel ill. So ideally, seek the help of a health professional, or at least do some additional research, before embarking on this type of treatment program.

Mold-killing agents include berberine, black seed, black walnut extract, cinnamon, coconut oil, colloidal silver, garlic, food-grade hydrogen peroxide, grapefruit seed extract, olive leaf extract, oregano oil, turmeric, and anti-fungal enzyme products. When such products are used, it is best to rotate them—using one agent for a month, then a different one the following month, and so on. This approach is required because some molds and fungi can adapt to a killing agent—rendering it less effective, if using the same remedy consistently.

For more information about mold in the body, have a read of my four-part blog called "The Real Cause of Alzheimer's Disease", on NutriStart's website. This blog series is based on a study examining 18 autopsied brains of Alzheimer patients, all contaminated with up to 10 different fungi. In these blogs I cover in detail how we pick up mold from our environment (e.g. washing machines), and our foods (e.g. approximately 25% of all grain crops are contaminate with mold, and toxic mold byproducts).

For those who are interested in finding out if they might have fungus in their brain, there is an online test, which can provide some clues. VCStest.com provides visual contrast sensitivity (VCS) testing to individuals who suffer (or suspect they may suffer) from a health condition which affects contrast sensitivity.

Visual contrast sensitivity testing measures one's ability to see details at low contrast levels, and is used as a (nonspecific) test of neurological function. A VCS test presents a series of images of decreasing contrast to the test subject, and records the contrast levels where patterns cannot be identified. The results of the test are used as an aid in the diagnosis of visual system dysfunction.

There are many things that can affect this ability to perceive contrast, including nutritional deficiencies, drug/medication use, exposure to neurotoxins and/or biotoxins, parasites, heavy metals, Lyme disease, and certain species of mold, and the mycotoxins they produce.

As mentioned, this test is considered nonspecific, thus VCS testing, by itself, is generally not diagnostic for any specific condition (including mold), but a positive result may suggest the existence of a health-affecting clinical, or subclinical, condition.

New accounts receive one free test initially, though free results are limited to a positive/negative determination, and raw test scores. If you need a detailed results interpretation, or if you want to test again, they request a small donation.

RESOURCES

Anti-EMF activist, Kim Goldberg, has a website devoted to personal stories, news items, and other information gathered while researching her book, "Refugium: Wi-Fi Exiles & The Coming Electroplague".

She is also collecting a list of "electro-safe" sanctuaries, and potential sanctuaries (still in the planning and fund-raising phase). For electro-hypersensitive people, moving to such sanctuaries may be necessary to survive—for others, simply taking a holiday in such a place, every once and a while, may be restorative.

This website (www.electroplague.com) includes links to other websites run by people who are currently forming EMF-free communities—buying land, looking for partners and funding, etc.—in various regions of North America. As well, the site contains links to Facebook groups that bring together people who want to create and/or share EMF-Free Sanctuaries:

- B.C. Wireless-Free Zones - www.facebook.com/groups/661015143934586/

- Wireless-Free Living Communities - www.facebook.com/groups/571481532909496/

A good, concise source of information on electrosensitivity can be found at www.weepinitiative.org, where, free of charge, you can read, or download, the booklet, "Living with Electrohypersensitivity: A Survival Guide". This Canadian website is also a valuable resource for those suffering from electrosensitivity, providing an information package that one can take to a doctor, if necessary.

Endnotes

1. Am J Epidemiol. 1979 Mar; 109(3):273-84; "Electrical wiring configurations and childhood cancer." Wertheimer N, Leeper E.
2. Left-sided Cancer: Blame your bed and TV? by R. Douglas Fields; Scientific American, July 2, 2010.

NUTRITIONAL PROTECTION FROM ELECTROSMOG

It seems counterintuitive to believe that something as nebulous as electromagnetic fields can damage us. And, stranger still to understand we can combat this insidiousness with nutrients. But, the fact is, much like with radiation, we can support the body in the areas that are most damaged by these modern assaults. EMFs, EMR, and RFs, all cause free radical damage, tear open cells (which makes them porous), damage DNA, and raise stress hormones.

Fortunately for us, even though much of the scientific community does not consider electrosmog to be a real danger, enough scientists have done studies on the subject to confirm there are measures we can take to protect ourselves. While most of these studies are animal and/or cultured-cell based, the research can be extrapolated to humans.

There are also some human studies that have been carried out—though they tend to observe only the damage these fields do, not how to counter that damage. Nevertheless, from this information we can move from determining, for example, that cell phone towers elevate cortisol levels in people who live near them, to discussing natural ways of lowering cortisol.

Now we will take a tour through the most researched foods, nutrients, and supplements, which work to protect our bodies from electromagnetic pollution.

MINERALS

Every cell in the body depends on minerals to perform its functions, and each cell acts like a biological battery. Essentially, minerals function as catalysts to keep these cellular batteries charged.

Without sufficient minerals, in the correct ratios, our cellular membranes cannot maintain the proper osmotic pressure between the inside and outside cell walls. That balanced pressure, along with maintaining the right pH, is what keeps viruses, and bacteria, from entering into cells. This internal cellular balance also protects cells from rupturing, preventing them from weakening and dying.

When cells are consistently exposed to high electromagnetic fields (including RF and EMR), a protective coating of calcium is removed from the cells, allowing them to rupture. Once ruptured, these cells lose their store of important minerals—most specifically calcium, copper, lithium, magnesium, potassium, and selenium.

Replacing these minerals is essential to maintaining good health, and combating the damaging effects of electrosmog. On a more basic level, minerals are alkalizing, and when dealing with any health issues (including gamma radiation), one of our most important defenses is to stay alkaline.

COPPER

Copper is necessary for protecting the myelin sheaths (an insulating layer of protein and fatty substances) which surround all of our nerves, including those in the brain, and spinal column. Myelin sheath damage is part of what causes Multiple Sclerosis, and since those so afflicted do not have the capacity to handle any more damage to their nervous systems, symptoms of MS (or any neurological condition) are worsened by exposure to electrosmog.

Copper deficiency also affects connective tissue, including collagen. Since electrosmog damages collagen (via increased cortisol levels), giving the body extra copper can be supportive of collagen production. Copper requires zinc (and vice versa), but both are usually found in a good multivitamin, or they can be purchased in a multi-mineral formula. Copper is generallytaken at a dose of 1 to 2 mg daily; any form of copper is fine, except copper sulfate (which can be toxic).

LITHIUM

Lithium, at high dosage levels, in the carbonate form, is used as a drug for treating bi-polar disorders, and, like any drug, can be dangerous, and have side effects. But, in small amounts, lithium is also a necessary trace mineral, very lacking in the modern diet. It protects neurons from radiation damage, and a deficiency is linked to Alzheimer's disease, anxiety, depression, drug addiction, violent crime, and suicide. As well, at low doses, in a natural form, lithium is a powerful mood elevator.

Lithium orotate is a commonly available supplement in the U.S. (and is the preferred form), but lithium supplements are not available to Canadians. As a supplement, to treat depression, and mild bipolar states, 10 mg of the orotate form is taken 1 to 3 times daily. For Canadians, the only legally available source, I am aware of, is "Concentrace Mineral Drops", which provides 1 mg of natural lithium per 40 drops (along with the full range of trace minerals). The seaweed, dulse, is also naturally high in lithium. An interesting fact about lithium—when the original 7-Up was launched, in 1929, it contained lithium as a medicinal, mood-boosting ingredient. It was later removed (in 1948) from the beverage.

MAGNESIUM

I have fully covered magnesium in another chapter, but here is yet another reason to ensure you provide your body with adequate levels. EMF exposure reduces magnesium levels, and since the body does not store magnesium (the way it stores calcium, and other minerals), it needs replenishing on a frequent basis.

Next to calcium, magnesium is the mineral found in the highest amounts in the cells, and, because it assists in the metabolism of calcium and potassium, magnesium is an important part of keeping cells resistant to electrosmog damage. Try to take 200 mg of supplemental magnesium twice daily, as a maintenance dose, and 300 mg twice daily if you are showing signs of magnesium deficiency.

POTASSIUM

Potassium deficiency causes muscle weakness, mental confusion, irregular heartbeat, adrenal and kidney problems, and edema. My friend, hypersensitive to EMFs, is constantly craving bananas, potatoes, fruit juice, and Low Sodium V8 (tomato juice cocktail)—all of which are extremely high in potassium.

In Canada, potassium supplements are a waste of time, since they are restricted to 99 mg, and we require around 4,000 mg daily. But, as indicated, there are many potassium-rich foods and beverages available, so, if you find yourself desiring any of them, you should indulge that craving. Other foods high in potassium include avocados, beans, dark leafy greens, fish, mushrooms, squash, tropical fruits, and yogurt.

SELENIUM

Selenium serves as an important component of our immune system, helping the body to make the master antioxidant, glutathione, and serving an anti-viral function. Selenium is also required in order to properly utilize iodine, which has a host of benefits, including protecting us from ionizing radiation, and preventing cancer growth.

One should try to ingest about 100 to 200 mcg of selenium daily, usually obtained through supplementation. In supplemental form, I prefer the yeast-derived selenium (e.g. SelenoExcell). If you take a multivitamin, be sure to check how much selenium it contains before buying an additional supplement, since most good multivitamins already contain between 100 and 200 mcg of selenium.

One can obtain relatively high amounts of selenium from eating Brazil nuts (2 nuts provides about 100 mcg), while other foods high in selenium include blue corn, sardines, garlic, lentils, onions, and nutritional yeast.

CALCIUM

I will go into much more detail about calcium, since its role is far more complicated than that of the other recently discussed minerals.

Constant exposure to electromagnetic pollution causes a loss of calcium, and excreting calcium can deposit in tissues, causing arthritis, and kidney stones, as well as contributing to osteoporosis, and pH imbalance. Adequate levels of calcium are also required for proper muscle contraction, and healthy moods.

Calcium ions help hold together the phospholipid molecules that are an essential part of the structure of cell membranes, and many studies have shown even weak electromagnetic fields remove calcium ions from cellular membranes, making them more likely to rupture and leak.

Although these tears in the cell wall can normally repair themselves, while the cell is open, and leaking, much damage can be done in the body. This mechanism alone can explain most of the ill effects caused by electromagnetic fields, since the cell membranes filter nutrients in and out of the cells, communicate with other cells, and regulate cell growth.

This theory of how electromagnetic fields cause illness, via calcium metabolism, was brought to the fore by Dr. Andrew Goldsworthy. He was the first to observe symptoms of electro-sensitivity were very similar to those caused by hypocalcemia (abnormally low calcium levels in the blood).

Dr. Goldsworthy theorized, if someone already has low levels of calcium in the blood, then exposure to EMFs—causing more calcium to leach from the cells—might be enough to push them over the edge.

Once pushed into the danger zone, by depletion of cellular and blood levels of calcium, one becomes victim to the symptoms of electro-sensitivity. Which happens to correspond with some of the acknowledged symptoms of hypocalcemia. These include cardiac arrhythmia, fatigue, gastro-intestinal ailments, muscle cramps, paresthesias (sensation of "pins and needles", or a burning feeling), and skin disorders.

Further symptoms attributed to electro-sensitivity, can be extrapolated from the effects of hypocalcemia. These include metabolic changes, cancer growth, genetic damage, infertility, immune suppression, inflammation, physiological stress responses, and negative effects on the brain. (1)

If you suspect you may be electro-sensitive, and/or have some of these symptoms, you can have your blood tested for ionized calcium levels. If the tests indicate abnormally low calcium levels, treating the hypocalcemia may relieve some, if not all, of these symptoms. A diagnosis of hypocalcemia is confirmed by the finding of a serum calcium level lower than 8.2 mg/dL (2.05 mmol/L), or an ionized calcium level lower than 4.4 mg/dL (1.1 mmol/L).

Following a diagnosis of hypocalcemia, medical professionals should then test for PTH (parathyroid hormone) levels. This test is required because hypocalcemia is most often caused by hypoparathyroidism.

In order to find the underlying cause of hypocalcemia, one will usually be tested for kidney function, as severe kidney malfunction can also be a cause. As well, one should have vitamin D, magnesium, and phosphate, levels checked. (Hypocalcemia can be caused by low vitamin D, and by extremely high or low magnesium, or phosphate, levels in the blood).

Certain drugs, such as bisphosphonates, diuretics, estrogen replacement therapy, fluorides, insulin, and excessive laxative use, can all also contribute to developing hypocalcemia.

The treatment for non-life threatening hypocalcemia is simply to take oral calcium supplements. However, calcium must be in balance with magnesium, for proper absorption, and to prevent magnesium deficiency from occurring.

Normally I do not recommend high levels of calcium, but, in this case, the recommendation is to take from 1,000 to 1,500 mg of elemental calcium per day (no more than 500 mg at a time). This should be accompanied by an amount of magnesium that is roughly half the amount of calcium (e.g. 500 mg of calcium, with 250 mg of magnesium, taken 2 or 3 times daily; skip weekends).

Some of the most absorbable forms of calcium are bisglycinate, citrate, coral, and mineralized algae. When symptoms abate, and blood tests confirm the situation has been rectified, I would suggest rolling back the dose to 250–300 mg of calcium (along with an equal amount of magnesium), twice daily. It is also important to take adequate amounts of vitamin D, which, once blood levels are normal, should be about 3,000–5,000 IU, taken five days a week.

VITAMIN D

Vitamin D is inescapably necessary as a supplement to ensure good health, but it also appears it may be especially important for people with electro-sensitivity. Professor Dominique Belpomme studied over 400 patients with electro-sensitivity, and found about 70% of them were deficient in vitamin D.

We already know vitamin D is neuro-protective, since chronic D-deficiency is linked to autism, Alzheimer's disease, dementia, depression, Parkinson's disease, and schizophrenia. Since many of the detrimental effects of electrosmog affect the brain, we can see why the neuro-protective attributes of vitamin D could be very important here. Vitamin D also helps to maintain serum calcium levels, so we have a second mechanism by which vitamin D can protect us from damaging electromagnetic fields.

EXAMINING ELECTROSENSITIVE HUMANS

Let's have a closer look at the work of Professor Belpomme, in part because these are not cultured cell, or rat, studies, but rather an examination of humans who are sensitive to EMFs. From May 2008 to March 2010, 425 patients who were hypersensitive to EMFs were examined in a clinical setting. Their responses to EMF exposure were divided into three phases.

In the first stage, EMF exposure induced some of these symptoms—headaches, a sensation of heating in the ear and/or the upper part of the body, tinnitus, visual abnormalities, muscle pain, dermatitis, chest tightness, palpitations, tachycardia, and/or nausea.

The second phase of exposure was characterized by symptoms of anxiety, attention deficit, behavioral problems, chronic fatigue, depression, insomnia, memory loss, and/or poor concentration. By the second phase, any of the first and second stage symptoms may occur every time the patient is exposed to EMFs.

The third phase, according to Professor Belpomme, occurs after long-term exposure, and, at least in electro-sensitive people, corresponds to a pre-Alzheimer's disease state. Professor Belpomme stated, "there is an important link between electromagnetic fields and neuro-degenerative diseases, notably Alzheimer's. The risk of Alzheimer's, which can arise in young persons from age 45, is moreover much more important than the risk of cancer".

Aside from discovering that 70% of these test subjects were deficient in vitamin D, Professor Belpomme and his team also discovered that 33% of them had decreased melatonin levels. Other aberrations observed included decreased blood flow in the limbic area of the brain, increased histamine levels in 36% of subjects, and an increase in "heat shock proteins" in 45% of them.

These "heat shock proteins" are also known as stress proteins, and an increase in their number is considered part of the stress response of an organism. Production of high levels of heat shock proteins can be triggered by exposure to different kinds of environmental stress conditions, such as infection, inflammation, exposure of the cell to toxins, starvation, and oxygen or water deprivation. The fact these stress indicators show up after exposure to electrosmog is further proof there is something dangerous going on here.

Elevated histamine levels (observed in this study) create increased vascular permeability, causing fluid to escape from capillaries into tissues, which lead to the standard symptoms of an allergic reaction: runny nose, watery eyes, itching, and/or sneezing. Histamine is also involved in regulating inflammatory and immune responses in the body. So increased histamine levels in electro-sensitive people can seriously aggravate allergy symptoms, and are an indication the immune system feels under attack.

What we can take away from this is more evidence of how damaging electromagnetic fields are to humans, and reasonable explanations of how they are linked to a variety of ailments.

Those who are hypersensitive to EMFs are going to show the outward symptoms more than those not hypersensitive. However, that does not mean the internal expressions of the ill effects (increased histamine, heat shock proteins, lowered levels of melatonin, etc), are not gradually weakening the bodies, and future health, of those seemingly untroubled by these electromagnetic fields.

At Professor Belpomme's clinic, the therapy for treating persons suffering from electromagnetic sensitivity includes prescriptions of Omega 3 fatty acids, antioxidants, vitamin D, and antihistamines. (2)

OMEGA-3 FATTY ACIDS

I am sure most of you reading this are well aware of the principles surrounding omega-3 essential fatty acids (EFAs), but I will briefly summarize for those who may not be as familiar.

While our bodies can make most of types of fatty acids it requires, from other fats and basic nutrients, this is not the case with omega-3 fatty acids. They are categorized as "essential" fatty acids because the body cannot make them from other elements, but must get them from food.

The foods highest in omega-3 fatty acids are deep-water fish, walnuts, and fresh ground flax seeds. From a supplemental approach, the prime sources of omega-3's are fish oils (caps or liquid), and flax seed oil (liquid, since you need 14 capsules to equal a tablespoon of oil).

There are now also concentrated algae-derived versions of omega-3, for vegetarians who want it in a capsule form, rather than taking flax oil by the tablespoon. These algae-based omega-3's are also available in liquid form, but require only a teaspoon-sized serving, being equal to fish oil in the amount of omega-3 they contain.

Professor Belpomme includes omega-3's as part of his protocol for electro-sensitive people because they are an integral part of cell membranes, and affect the function of cell receptors in these membranes. As we saw in the section on calcium, the rupturing of cell membranes is one of the underlying reasons why EMFs are damaging to our health. So, anything that helps stabilize that membrane, will help protect us against electrosmog.

Omega 3 fatty acids are also involved in making hormones that regulate blood clotting and inflammation, and they also bind to receptors in cells that regulate genetic function. Since EMF damage can involve increased inflammatory markers, increased platelet clumping in the blood, and DNA damage, we can see other protective effects of omega 3's that directly relate to the issue at hand.

The standard recommendation for supplementing with omega 3 EFAs is 1000 mg of total EPA and DHA (not just a 1000 mg capsule of fish oil), or 1 tablespoon of flax oil, per day. However, much higher doses are used to treat certain ailments, including neurological conditions (MS, Parkinson's disease, ALS, etc.). Also, those in poor health (neurological conditions, diabetes, thyroid disorders) may have a hard time converting flax oil into DHA and EPA, as do vegans (possibly because they are missing some essential nutrients). Therefore, if you are electro-sensitive, you may find it beneficial to ensure you are obtaining preformed omega 3 from fish, or algae, and not relying exclusively on flax oil.

One other highly absorbable form of omega 3 is krill oil, which requires only 1500 mg per day to be clinically effective, versus 3,000 to 5,000 mg (or more) of regular fish oil. Because krill oil exists in a "phospholipid" form, rather than in a "triglyceride" form, as with other fish oils, it enters into the cells of the body far more easily than conventional fish oils.

ANTIOXIDANTS

Supplementing with antioxidants is another part of the protocol at Professor Belpomme's clinic. Studies show even low frequency EMFs reduce levels of antioxidants in our bodies, resulting in free radical damage to our cells, and DNA. The antioxidants most suppressed by EMF exposure are melatonin, vitamin C, vitamin E, superoxide dismutase (SOD), and glutathione.

At the time of this writing, eight rodent studies exist that show vitamins C and E, along with melatonin, protect against damage caused by cell phone emissions. These nutrients particularly target the oxidative stress (free radical damage) caused by electromagnetic pollution, which is related to increased cancer risk.

In one of these studies, the rat subjects were divided into groups: one group received electromagnetic radiation exposure, but no antioxidants; the other groups receiving treatment with melatonin only, vitamin C only, or vitamins C and E only, before exposure to EMR (and a control group, which did not receive radiation or any treatment).

After the treatment period (from 10 to 30 days), scientists found endometrial (lining of the uterus) damage, fibrosis, kidney damage, skin changes, and oxidative stress, in the animals who received EMR exposure only. Yet, these negative effects were reversed in the groups receiving melatonin along with vitamins C and E. (3)

It appears that vitamin C protected the aqueous (or watery) areas of the cell, while vitamin E protected the fatty areas of the cell—which makes sense, since vitamin C is a water-soluble nutrient, and vitamin E is a fat-soluble one. Since the fatty area of the cell includes the cell membrane, vitamin E will clearly help prevent the aforementioned leakage from cells that EMR induces, and may therefore also help protect nerve membranes.

Another two of the eight rat studies showed that melatonin significantly protected against retinal (eye), and kidney damage, caused by cell phone radiation, when compared to subjects that did not receive melatonin. (4) (5)

Standard recommendation for supplementing with vitamin C is to take 500 to 1000 mg, three times daily, though much higher amounts are used therapeutically. It is recommended to take 400 to 800 IU of natural source vitamin E daily ("mixed" vitamin E), with a meal containing fat. Though, again, higher doses can be taken for therapeutic purposes, with the advice of a health professional.

GLUTATHIONE

As we have seen, powerful antioxidants are our first line of defense against electromagnetic-induced free radical damage to our cells. Glutathione is our most powerful, internally generated antioxidant, and also is an important part of the detoxification process. So maintaining high levels of glutathione is one of the best things we can do to protect ourselves from modern dangers.

Certain foods help the body produce glutathione by providing the necessary building block, which is sulfur. The mineral sulfur is found in fish, grass-fed beef, free-range poultry and eggs, and in many plant foods, including chives, garlic, leeks, onions, and shallots.

As well as the onion family, the cruciferous vegetable family also contains high amounts of sulfur compounds (in this case known as glucosinolates). These include arugula, bok choy, broccoli, Brussels sprouts, cabbage, cauliflower, collard greens, horseradish, kale, mustard, radish, rutabaga, turnips, wasabi, and watercress. As a bonus, some studies have shown that high intakes of cruciferous vegetables are associated with a lower risk of lung, and colorectal, cancer.

The food that contains the most preformed glutathione is asparagus, which also contains a good amount of selenium. Asparagus is particularly good for the kidneys (which are often damaged by electrosmog), and is even used as an alternative cancer treatment. The other food highest in glutathione is avocado.

It is important to note the sulfur content of soil influences the sulfur concentrations found in plants, so all recommended foods are most valuable when they are organically grown.

Other supplements that elevate glutathione levels are vitamin C (500 mg minimum), milk thistle (250–500 mg standardized extract, taken 1 to 3 times daily), and whey protein (concentrate or isolate).

A few other supplements will also raise glutathione levels, but with these, more care must be taken, since some animal studies indicate they can also bind to mercury, and redistribute it back to the nervous system. These are N-acetyl L-cysteine (NAC), alpha lipoic acid (R+ALA), and acetyl-L-carnitine (ALC).

Thus, if you know you have a high load of mercury in your system (or even if you just have mercury dental fillings), you should use caution when taking these particular supplements, or seek advice from a health professional.

There is one form of carnitine that can be used even by those with mercury toxicity. While acetyl-L-carnitine is a form of carnitine that works on the brain—increasing neurotransmitter levels—simple L-carnitine does not go into the brain, and so is safer to use for those with high mercury levels.

L-carnitine is an amino acid found only in animal proteins (and thus can be lacking in a strict vegetarian diet). It strengthens the heart muscle, and is used to aid in weight loss programs, since it shuttles fat from the blood into the mitochondria, to be burned as fuel for the body.

Furthermore, there is a study showing L-carnitine, when combined with selenium, elevated glutathione levels in animals subjected to EMF stress.

In this study, animals exposed to electromagnetic fields were found to have lower levels of antioxidants (vitamins A, C and E), in their blood than a group not exposed to the fields. In the experimental group, given selenium and L-carnitine, concentrations of vitamins A, C, and E, were higher, and the activity of glutathione peroxidase was much higher, than in a group exposed to the electromagnetic field, but given no treatment. As well, lipid peroxidation levels in irradiated animals treated with selenium and L-carnitine were lower than in those exposed to irradiation, but given no supplementation—indicating a protective action on the cells. (6)

L-carnitine is usually taken at a dose of 500 –1000 mg, one to three times daily on an empty stomach.

ROSMARINIC ACID

Rosmarinic acid (RA) belongs to the class of micronutrients known as polyphenols. Like most polyphenols it has antioxidant, anti-allergic, anti-carcinogenic, anti-inflammatory, antiviral, and antimicrobial properties. Because the antioxidant activity of RA is even stronger than that of vitamin E, and because of its antibacterial properties, it is often used as a natural preservative for foods, and cosmetics.

Technically a phenolic acid, rosmarinic acid was given its name because it was first discovered hiding in the herb rosemary. Rosmarinic acid is an ester of caffeic acid and 3, 4-dihydroxyphenyllactic acid, which I only mention because we will be discussing caffeic acid shortly.

As far as serving as a protective nutrient against electrosmog, we have yet another rat study, backed up by the already determined fact that RA works to prevent free radical damage to cell membranes. As we have seen earlier, damage to cell membranes is one of the major side effects of electrosmog, so anything that helps to prevent that tearing of the membrane is of value here.

The objective of this rat study was to observe the effect of RA on sertoli cell (part of male fertility) apoptosis (death), and serum antioxidant levels in rats, after being exposed to electromagnetic fields.

The conclusion arrived at was, "Level of testosterone, total antioxidant capacity, significantly increased in groups that received rosmarinic acid. Since in our study 5mg/rat of rosmarinic acid showed a significantly preventive effect on cell damage, especially sertoli cells apoptosis that is caused by EMF exposure, it seems that using rosmarinic acid as food additive can be effective for supporting people living under EMF environmental pollution." (7)

Here we see RA both mitigated free radical damage done to cells exposed to electrosmog, and compensated for the damage to fertility these fields cause (by naturally elevating testosterone levels).

Since we have already discussed how electromagnetic fields increase the growth, virulence, and amount of mold in buildings, it is good news to find that RA also has some benefit in this department. Two common mycotoxins (dangerous mold byproducts) were studied to find out how RA might fare against them.

Aflatoxin B (found in peanuts, cornmeal, cooking oils, and milk from cows fed moldy grains), and ochratoxin A (found in coffee, grain, pork, grapes, heating ducts, and water-damaged houses), both cause oxidative damage, compromise liver function, and are considered to be seriously carcinogenic.

In this study, RA reduced free radical production, DNA synthesis inhibition, and cell death, caused by the mycotoxins. Since we know that electrosmog also causes free radical damage, cell death, and inhibits DNA repair, all these benefits of RA apply equally to preventing the dangers electrosmog. (8)

Rosmarinic acid is easily absorbed from the intestinal tract—meaning it is effective when consumed in foods, or taken in supplement form. It naturally occurs at relatively high levels in many plants, and in fact, it turns out that rosemary is not even the highest source of RA. One analysis of rosemary for its RA content found that the level varied widely, and depended on several factors including climate, soil conditions, harvest time, and storage conditions.

Researchers analyzed a variety of plants, from a number of different countries, in order to find those that are the best consistent sources of RA. Compared to rosemary the following plants were consistently higher in RA: Salvia officinalis (common or garden sage), Melissa officinalis (lemon balm), Thymus citriodorous (lemon thyme), and Mentha spicata (spearmint). (9)

Other plants naturally high in RA include common basil, Holy Basil, fennel, peppermint, thyme, and the herb "self-heal" (Prunella vulgaris).

BASIL

While common basil (Ocimum basilicum) did not show up in the above list of the highest sources of RA, it still comes in as a reasonably high source of the substance. It also has its own studies showing protection against EMF-induced free radical damage, and cell death.

As we have established, damage to cells caused by the oxidative stress of prolonged exposure to EMR, causes cells to rupture and die. Our first line of defense is the powerful free radical scavenging enzymes produced by the body (catalase, SOD, and glutathione).

Common basil has been used medicinally for centuries, in China, and India, and its antioxidant benefits are already well known to Western science. As a result, scientists hypothesized this herb might also protect ovarian tissue from reactive oxygen species (a form of free radical). In this study, rats exposed to EMFs for 40 consecutive days, were supplemented with basil extract (1.5g/kg). The group given basil extract showed significantly higher levels of SOD than the control group.

This study "demonstrated that the administration of Ocimum basilicum can overcome reproductive toxicity of EMF effects. In conclusion this natural extract (Ocimum basilicum) as an anti-oxidant can protect ovary tissue and follicles and it is also able to reduce apoptosis in ovary tissue". These results confirm similar experiments done with basil, and other RA containing herbs. (10)

Basil can be eaten as a spice (found in pesto, and other sauces), but is not commonly available as a supplement. However, Holy Basil is available in supplement form, and has most of the same antioxidant properties as common basil, with even stronger benefits for mood enhancement, and cortisol lowering.

CAFFEIC ACID

Caffeic acid, and its derivative caffeic acid phenethyl ester (CAPE), are produced in many kinds of plants. To some degree, caffeic acid (CA) is present in all plants, since it is used by plants to produce lignin—an integral part of the secondary cell walls of plants. CA has proven itself a powerful antioxidant, also showing anti-inflammatory activity, and the ability to regulate the immune system.

As we saw in the chapter on Electrosmog, one of the worst health issues raised by this new form of pollution is the rise in toxic mold levels in buildings, and homes. Research done at the United States Department of Agriculture showed CA to be the most effective natural substance for reducing aflatoxin production in plants, reducing levels by 95%. As a result, their scientists recommended it be used as a natural fungicide, to protect trees and plants. (11)

Caffeic acid is found at relatively high levels in a number of consumable plants, as well as in the oil produced from the kernels of the argan tree. While argan oil is mostly used for cosmetic purposes here in the West, in Morocco, argan oil is used to dip bread in, and is used on couscous, pasta, or salad. There, argan oil is considered to help prevent cancer, heart disease, and obesity.

Some of the best sources of CA are asparagus, barley, cabbage, olives, olive oil, spinach, white grapes, and white wine. The herb echinacea purpurea is also high in CA, and is known to exert a protective effect against cellular damage caused by exposure to ionizing radiation.

CAPE

As mentioned above, a derivative of CA is caffeic acid phenethyl ester (CAPE), and this component has an even more specific action against electrosmog. One study aimed to "investigate the possible protective effects of caffeic acid phenethyl ester (CAPE) on lipid peroxidation (LPO) and the activities of antioxidant enzymes in the livers of rats exposed to the 900 MHz electromagnetic field (EMF)".

The researchers were well aware of how electromagnetic pollution from cell phones increased free radical damage, which leads to lipid peroxidation—a process in which free radicals "steal" electrons from the lipids in cell membranes, resulting in cell damage. They were also looking to see if they could prevent the liver from having its antioxidant producing abilities inhibited.

This study used CAPE extracted from propolis, since "several studies suggest that supplementation with antioxidants can influence EMF exposure induced hepatotoxicity" (liver damage). CAPE naturally occurs, in high amounts, in bee propolis—a resinous substance collected by bees from the buds of various trees—used as a sealant in the construction of hives. Propolis is highly antimicrobial, protecting the hive from bacterial infection, and has been used by humans for centuries to fight infection, and support immune function.

While levels of liver-produced antioxidants (SOD and glutathione) were clearly reduced in the rats exposed to 900 MHz EMFs, animals receiving the CAPE supplement saw levels of those antioxidant compounds increase. Therefore, "It can be concluded that

CAPE may prevent the 900 MHz EMF-induced oxidative changes in liver by strengthening the antioxidant defense system by reducing reactive oxygen species and increasing antioxidant enzyme activities". (12)

The product used in this test is now on the market (though I have yet to see it in Canada). Known as "Capolis", it is the first naturally derived form of caffeic acid phenethyl ester, and is standardized to contain 5% CAPE. Capolis has proven itself a powerful antioxidant and anti-inflammatory—even protecting the brain from inflammation. (www.capolis.com) If one cannot find this particular product, propolis liquid, and capsules, are commonly available at health food stores.

CHLOROGENIC ACID

Though caffeic acid (CA) is unrelated to caffeine, it is found (naturally occurring) in coffee. In coffee, and many other types of fruits, caffeic and quinic acid combine to form chlorogenic acid. Coffee is one of the highest sources of chlorogenic acid—even more so when the beans are green—which is why green coffee bean extracts are marketed for weight loss, insulin regulation, and cholesterol control. All such benefits stem from the chlorgenic acid.

The fruits highest in chlorogenic acid are apples, blueberries, cherries, kiwis, pears, and plums, though the major source in the modern diet is coffee. Coffee drinkers average 0.5 to 1 gram, per day, whereas those who do not drink coffee usually get less than 100 mg. It should be pointed out that, while the absorption of caffeic acid from food is around 95%, the absorption of chlorogenic acid appears to be about 33%. Nonetheless, there are many other benefits to be gained from eating the above-mentioned foods.

GINGKO

Ginkgo biloba is a well-researched herb, known for its support of mental functions, including cognition, memory, and mood. Now a new study has shown gingko can also protect against oxidative stress to the brain caused by cell phone radiation.

In this study, rats were exposed to 900 MHz electromagnetic radiation from cell phones for 7 days (for only 1 hour a day). Results clearly showed evidence of oxidative damage from this EMR exposure, but much of the damage was prevented with the administration of ginkgo. In this case, ginkgo appeared to work by helping to preserve antioxidant enzyme activity in brain tissue. (13)

The standard dose for gingko is 60 mg, three times daily, with most clinical studies based on using a standardized extract of ginkgo (24% flavone glycosides, 6% terpene lactones). Cheap gingko supplements have proven to be of little value, while clinically proven products have shown to have a wide range of additional benefits—including treating erectile dysfunction, and circulatory disorders. Two clinically tested products are Ginkgold from Nature's Way, and Gingko products produced by A. Vogel.

GREEN TEA

Green tea is an amazing substance, pretty much protecting us from everything dangerous to our health. It is anti-inflammatory, anti-carcinogenic, antibacterial, antiviral, antifungal, and is an antioxidant. It is protective against both gamma radiation (ionizing radiation) and electromagnetic radiation (non-ionizing radiation).

One study was designed to investigate the potential protective effects of green tea polyphenols, against electromagnetic radiation-induced injury, in cultured rat cortical neurons (brain cells in a petri dish). Here, green tea polyphenols were used to treat the cultured cortical neurons (which had been exposed to 1800 MHz EMR from a cell phone), and the conclusion was positive: "Our results suggested a neuroprotective effect of green tea polyphenols against the mobile phone irradiation-induced injury on the cultured rat cortical neurons." (14)

Green tea should be organic to get the full benefits, and these benefits accrue at 3 to 5 cups per day. Taking green tea orally (as a liquid) has three advantages over swallowing it in capsule form: it prevents the bacteria that cause bad breath, works to prevent cavities, and protects against oral cancer.

MISCELLANEOUS

Methylcobalamin (B-12), and folic acid (ideally, in the methylfolate form), are required for a healthy nervous system, and to prevent neurological disorders. Many of the B vitamins are also necessary for the production of neurotransmitters, including B-3 for serotonin, and B-6 for dopamine production. Pantothenic Acid (B-5) is necessary to support the adrenal glands, helping to keep cortisol in check. Therefore, one should not overlook the basic B-complex (or a multivitamin that contains the B-complex vitamins), when putting together a regimen to help cope with the negative effects of electrosmog.

Alternative medicines, such as acupressure, acupuncture, and Qigong (pronounced chi gong), may provide some benefits for those who are electro-sensitive. Acupressure, and acupuncture, therapies are based on the assumption that humans have electrical channels called meridians. Therefore, the therapeutic use of acupuncture, or acupressure, may be helpful to rebalance our delicate electrical system, after interference from external sources of disruptive electrical frequencies.

Microwaves increase free radicals via the "iron-catalyzed Fenton cycle". Therefore, iron, in its unbound form (as a supplement), may be undesirable for those with electro-sensitivity, who live near cell phone towers. Determining if iron is going to be a problem is something such people will have to monitor. If you have electrosensitivity, track how you feel (better or worse), while taking an iron supplement. Even so, only take iron if you have reason to believe you may be deficient. Iron supplementation is not recommended for men (unless they are vegetarian), or women past menstruation (unless vegetarian), except in cases of diagnosed anemia.

The presence of metal implants within tissue, or even metal worn on the body, may result in excess electromagnetic exposure, due to metal's ability to absorb and retain electromagnetic energy. So, if you are electro-sensitive, it may be advisable to minimize the use of metal implants, metal-rimmed eyeglasses, metal wires in orthodontic braces, and the wearing of metallic objects, such as belt buckles and jewelry.

Some have found that silver-mercury amalgam fillings can cause a worsening of symptoms, and that (safely performed) mercury removal helps to alleviate symptoms. It also appears that simply having high levels of mercury (and other heavy metals) in the body can also make one more sensitive to EMFs. Essentially, the metals in the body, and blood, act as an antenna, picking up and storing electromagnetic charges. Heavy metal detoxification then becomes a necessity for these people, if other related health issues have not already made that apparent.

A good naturopath can help with testing for heavy metal levels in the body, and with a regimen to remove them. Currently one of the most effective methods of removing heavy metals is the infrared sauna (while doing a small amount of exercise before, along with ingesting niacin (B-3) to the flush-point).

Moving mercury out of the body must be done delicately, as one can simply move mercury out of storage (from fat cells), and allow it to roam in the body, settling in areas where it can do more damage (like the brain) than if it had been left alone. Do not attempt mercury detoxification on your own unless you do a lot of research first.

Endnotes

1. "The Biological Effects of Weak Electromagnetic Fields"; Andrew Goldsworthy, 2007; www.es-uk.info.

2. Presentation of Prof. Dominique Belpomme at 8th National Congress on Electrosmog, Berne, 2011: www.weepnews.blogspot.ca; "The Canadian Initiative to Stop Wireless, Electric, and Electromagnetic Pollution."

3. Oral B, et al. Endometrial apoptosis induced by a 900-MHz mobile phone: preventive effects of vitamins E and C. Adv Ther. 2006 Nov-Dec; 23(6):957-73.

4. Ozguner F, et al. "Comparative analysis of the protective effects of melatonin and caffeic acid phenethyl ester (CAPE) on mobile phone-induced renal impairment in rat." Mol Cell Biochem. 2005 Aug; 276(1-2):31-7.

5. Ozguner F, et al. Protective effects of melatonin and caffeic acid phenethyl ester against retinal oxidative stress in long-term use of mobile phone: a comparative study. Mol Cell Biochem. 2006 Jan; 282(1-2):83-8.

6. "Selenium and L-Carnitine Reduce Oxidative Stress in the Heart of Rat Induced by 2.45-GHz Radiation from Wireless Devices." Turker Y, et al. Published in: Biol Trace Elem Res 2011.

7. Afr J Tradit Complement Altern Med. 2013 Oct 3; 10(6):477-80. "Effect of rosmarinic acid on sertoli cells apoptosis and serum antioxidant levels in rats after exposure to electromagnetic fields." Hajhosseini L, et al.

8. "Effects of rosmarinic acid against aflatoxin B1 and ochratoxin-A-induced cell damage in a human hepatoma cell line (Hep G2)"; J Appl Toxicol. 2004.

9. Pharmacogn Mag. 2012 Jan-Mar; 8 (29): 37–41. "Comparative study of rosmarinic acid content in some plants of Labiatae family."; Maryam Shekarchi, et al.

10. Arash Khaki, et al. "Effect of Ocimum basilicum on Ovary tissue Apoptosis after exposed with extremely low frequency electromagnetic fields (ELF-EMF) in Rats." Life Sci J; 2013.

11. USDA Agricultural Research Service; Bruce C. Campbell and Jong H. Kim; Plant Mycotoxin Research Unit at ARS's Western Regional Research Center in Albany, CA.

12. Toxicol Ind Health. 2009 Jul; 25(6):429-34; "The protective effect of caffeic acid phenethyl ester (CAPE) on oxidative stress in rat liver exposed to the 900 MHz electromagnetic field." Koyu A, et al.

13. Ilhan A, et al; "Ginkgo biloba prevents mobile phone-induced oxidative stress in rat brain." Clin Chim Acta. 2004 Feb; 340(1-2):153-62.

14. Neurotox Res. 2011 Oct; 20(3):270-6. "Potential protection of green tea polyphenols against 1800 MHz electromagnetic radiation-induced injury on rat cortical neurons." Liu ML, et al.

DIRTY ELECTRICITY AND GEOPATHIC STRESS

There are two more types of dangerous magnetic fields to be aware of, but don't be discouraged; these are the last two. One is natural, known as geopathic stress, and the other is man-made, and referred to as dirty electricity. Let's begin with the latter.

DIRTY ELECTRICITY

You can protect your home with anti-EMF technologies, and switch from wireless to hard-wired connections, but if you have dirty electricity running through your household wiring, emitting electrical pollution, your health can still be adversely affected.

What I am technically referring to when I say dirty electricity is actually a form of electromagnetic pollution—also known as electromagnetic interference (EMI), or high-frequency voltage transients. Dirty electricity is caused by high frequency electrical energy, traveling through the wiring in buildings where only standard household currents (60-Hertz AC) should be.

Any device that interrupts the 60-Hertz current flow will generate dirty electricity because each interruption of current flow results in a voltage spike—causing EMF surges to occur in the building. Thus, whenever modern appliances, energy-efficient lights, or virtually any other kind of "new and improved" electronic technology, converts standard 60-Hertz AC electricity into other forms of electricity, the result is constant low-level EMF pollution.

For example, energy efficient compact fluorescent bulbs operate in a range as high as 100 kHz, and for these bulbs to function, the household current has to be boosted. This charge can then contaminate the wiring in your house, even if it does not occur from within your dwelling, since all homes, in essence, share the same wiring (issuing from the electrical provider).

Here are some of the other worst producers of dirty electricity in homes, and offices: computers, DC chargers, dimmer switches, regular fluorescent lighting, printers, transmitters, variable speed motors, and smart meters.

Cell phone towers are especially bad for dumping dirty electricity back into the shared electrical grid. These towers have to switch power supplies, in order to convert the alternating current (AC) from the electrical grid into direct current (DC). This is necessary in order to operate the tower transmitter, and to keep the batteries charged (required for backup power, in event of a power outage).

Because much of dirty electricity is in the radio frequency (RF) range, it radiates electromagnetic fields several feet from the wall (where the wiring is) even when electrical devices are off. Dirty electricity will spread throughout a building, and to other buildings, by way of electrical wiring, ground/plumbing currents, and power lines.

Studies performed in schools and libraries indicated dirty electricity causes increased rates of cancer, and hyperactivity. For an overview of these studies, along with information on how these ailments can be turned around by using Graham Stetzer (GS) filters, see the article, "Dirty electricity, chronic stress, neurotransmitters and disease," by Samuel Milham and David Stetzer—available at www.dirtyelectricity.org. Another informative website is www.dirtyelectricity.ca, which also provides information on how to use a Graham Stetzer meter, and the proper way to use GS filters. Also highly recommended, as a source for dirty electricity filters, is www.greenwavefilters.com.

ELECTRICITY IN THE GOOD OLD DAYS

Epidemiological evidence links dirty electricity to most of the "diseases of civilization", including ADHD, cancer, cardiovascular disease, diabetes, and suicide—all of which began to increase at the turn of the twentieth century. This is a fascinating theory, implying we have always suffered from overexposure to electromagnetic fields—long before other forms of electrosmog existed.

Electrification of residences occurred gradually, over the first few decades of the 20th century. By the 1940s, there was a clear distinction between those who lived in urban areas, with nearly full electrification of homes, and those in rural areas, who were mostly non-electrified. In the U.S., census records exist covering the period from 1920 to 1960, as the process of electrification slowly spread across America, moving from the cities to incorporate the countryside.

Researcher Samuel Milhamemail decided to compare urban and rural death rates, and correlate them with electrification rates for the decade of 1940. He discovered cities had much higher levels of death by modern disease (and suicide), than did non-electrified rural areas.

His conclusion was, "I hypothesize that the 20th century epidemic of the so called diseases of civilization including cardiovascular disease, cancer and diabetes and suicide was caused by electrification not by lifestyle. A large proportion of these diseases may therefore be preventable". (Historical evidence that electrification caused the 20th century epidemic of "diseases of civilization". Samuel Milhamemail; Washington State Department of Health, Olympia, WA, USA; August 18, 2009)

Yet, it is not as though the dangers of over-exposure to electromagnetic fields only appeared in hindsight, gradually coming to light by way of studies like these. Awareness of the unhealthy nature of this early form of electrosmog showed up at the turn of the 20th century, among telegraph line installers, and telephone switchboard operators.

Switchboard operators were exposed to hundreds of live telephone connections every working day, along with the electromagnetic fields that radiated from their headsets. The link between ailments and the job was so obvious that, in 1907, Bell switchboard operators in Toronto went on strike, demanding shorter working hours, and safer working conditions.

In the 1950s, radar operators who worked near large radar antennas reported a range of symptoms, referred to at that time as radio wave, or microwave, illness. Symptoms experienced by these early victims of EMFs included anxiety, convulsions, depression, fatigue, nerve damage, and rashes, among others. (All symptoms reported currently, by those who are electrosensitive.)

Regardless of whether or not we work in jobs that involve high-level exposure to EMFs, we are all suffering from chronic exposure these days.

For the full story on this early example of damage caused by EMF exposure, go to www.magdahavas.com. This website also offers both Canadian, and international, information on electrosensitivity, information on what you can do personally and politically, and up-to-date news stories on the issue.

GEOPATHIC STRESS

Even before the advent of electricity, our ancestors had their own energy problems—now known as geopathic stress. Geopathic stress refers to "bad" earth energies, which can adversely affect health. In the past, most cultures had an awareness of geopathic stress zones; for example, in Feng Shui, the Chinese referred to geopathic stress by many names, including "claws of the dragon", or "dragon lines."

While this subject is well understood in China, and Europe, it is less known in North America, and falls outside the domain of modern science. Nonetheless, I will touch briefly on the subject, and if you feel you have covered all your electronic bases, and still suspect your home of making you ill, I suggest you do further research into the subject of geopathic stress. (For more information visit www. geopathology.com.)

Geopathic stress occurs when the natural radiation that rises up through the earth (the Schumann resonance), becomes distorted, or disrupted, by weak electromagnetic fields. These fields are created by underground streams, certain mineral concentrations, geological fault lines, and underground cavities. Making matters worse are human alterations of the landscape, including underground cables, sewage lines, water pipes, tunnels, and road construction projects— all of which can cause or intensify geopathic stress.

SYMPTOMS OF GEOPATHIC STRESS

Farming communities have long known that building a barn over an underground stream will lead to poor milk production, and an increase in miscarriages in cows. This same negative energy will also cause ill health in humans: chronic exposure to geopathic stress can negatively affect mood and energy levels, as well as weaken the immune system. Those working or sleeping in areas with high geopathic stress often complain of feeling listless and drained, sometimes to the point of experiencing chronic fatigue.

Other symptoms linked to geopathic stress include chronic inflammation, headaches, heart problems, infertility, irritability, miscarriages, and disturbed sleep patterns (including frequent nightmares). Geopathic stress is also linked to behavioral problems in children, including attention deficit disorder, bedwetting, hyperactivity, incessant crying, and learning disorders.

Furthermore, high geopathic stress zones create a greater susceptibility to bacteria, parasites, and viruses, along with a compromised immune system—all of which conspire to cause a wide range of serious health issues. According to experts in the field, these issues can include cancerous tumors, leukemia, lymphoma, and neurological problems.

There are a few strong clues indicating geopathic stress may be a problem in your home. One clue is, you never wake up feeling refreshed, and in fact, actually feel worse in the mornings. Another is, just a feeling there is something wrong with your home—somehow, it doesn't feel right, you don't look forward to going home, and you feel better when you are not at home. Supporting this feeling would be the knowledge that previous occupants of your house had experienced cancer, or other serious illnesses.

Finally, if you have a serious ailment not responding to treatment, or it is one ailment after another, for no understandable reasons, you may be dealing with a high geopathic stress environment. For more clues, a geopathic stress questionnaire is available at www.helios3.com.

DETECTING GEOPATHIC STRESS

Geopathic stress cannot be detected with conventional EMF testing devices—instead, it is usually discovered by "dowsing", with pendulums, or dowsing rods. This means you will need to find a dowsing expert in your area, if you want to check for this form of energy pollution—or learn to dowse yourself (lessons available on YouTube). Lest you think this is hokum, know that to this day (even in the West) people seek the services of a dowser in order to determine the best place to drill a water-well.

There is however at least one device I found that claims to detect geopathic stress areas. This German instrument (developed by Dr. Ernst Hartmann and Dr. Dieter Ashcroft), is called the Genitron Felix-3, and is used in German universities and research institutes.

In ancient Europe, before building a house or barn, sheep were sent to graze in the area in question—where the sheep chose to sleep was then determined to be a safe place to build. Sheep, like most mammals, instinctively avoid high geopathic stress areas. Other mammals particularly sensitive to damage done by geopathic stress are dogs, cattle, and horses. If you have any of these animals, and they are often agitated for no apparent reason, escape frequently, will not bed in a fixed place, are infertile, or often ill, you may wish to have their sleeping area (or barn) tested for these energies.

Some creatures actually prefer high geopathic stress areas. These include ants, bees, cats, owls, slugs, snails, snakes, and wasps. Interestingly, bees will actually produce more honey when located in a geopathic stress zone, so while this energy is clearly not good for humans, it does have its purpose in life.

When observing locations that a cat may like, we do have to take into account they are often just drawn to a warm and cozy place. So, simply noting a cat's favorite spot, may not be enough information to determine a high stress zone. However, if the cat always chooses the same spot on the bed, and if one's health is not good, this may be an important clue. It can also be helpful to just be aware the areas which the cat prefers, are worse for you to spend time in, than the areas preferred by the dog.

Many plants also like geopathic stress areas, including docks, ferns, foxglove, ivy, lichen, elderberry trees, moss, nettles, night-shades, and thistles.

It has been observed that this natural form of radiation, like man-made electromagnetic fields, also encourages mold to grow. Therefore, beer, cheese, fruit, jam, vegetables, wine, and even photographic film, will all spoil unusually fast, when stored in a geopathic stress zone.

Other vegetation-related clues to stress zones include lighting-struck trees, infertile fruit trees (fruit trees are the most sensitive of the tree family), dead or stunted gaps in hedges or avenues of trees, and unnaturally twisted trees. Lawns will show bare patches, moss, and fungi, while vegetable gardens will produce stunted, or mutated, plants.

Observing any of these plants, or aforementioned creatures, in a given area, can be a clue that geopathic stress may be present. As well, an anthill in your yard, or moss on your lawn (moss indicating water flowing underground), can also indicate you may have these energies affecting your dwelling.

Further clues include, paths of chronically unresolved clutter within the home, cracks in glass, brick or plasterwork, piles of debris, recurring mechanical and electrical breakdowns, derelict areas, and accident spots both within the home and outside. Road accidents will happen more often in geopathic stress zones—in fact in some countries, these roads will have warning signs—and such roads are more prone to developing potholes.

Some of the plants found in geopathic stress zones have medicinal properties, including nettles, foxglove, and elderberry. Thus, it is no surprise that geopathic practitioners believe the appropriate herbs for treating an ailment caused by geopathic stress, are often found growing in the same area. For example, if one were suffering from viral conditions, they could use the antiviral properties of elderberry to treat their condition.

PROTECTING AGAINST GEOPATHIC STRESS

Protecting your habitat against geopathic stress will most likely require the help of a specialist as, again, it falls outside the reach of modern science. Dowsers will re-route, or weaken, geopathic stress, by burying metal rods outside, and/or placing copper coils over problematic areas in the house (hidden under carpet or shelving, or located in the attic or basement). One thing that evidently interrupts the flow of geopathic energy is cork, so people will often place cork tiles under their bed to protect that most important area. Sometimes, simply moving the bed to another area of the bedroom can make a big difference.

There is an effective homeopathic product, called Geovita, that helps the body cope with geopathic stress, and also treats sensitivity to electrosmog. It is available through homeopaths, naturopaths, or at www.biomedicine.com.

As mentioned in the chapter, Protection from Electrosmog, one helpful device is Total Shield, which also generates an electromagnetic field that mimics the Earth's natural frequency (the Schumann Resonance). The designers of this product claim this frequency will neutralize much of the damage caused by geopathic stress. The Total Shield starts at $400 US (for the basic model), and is available from www.brimhall.com. There are also cheaper devices available, which reproduce only the Schumann Resonance. (www.schumannresonator.com)

Other devices claiming to neutralize the ill effects of geopathic stress—utilizing Multi-Wave Oscillators, or Radionics, to accomplish this—include, the Spiral Of Tranquillity (www.lessstress.ie), Helios 3 (www.helios3.com), and Geomack machines (www.geomack.com).

CONCLUSION

One final note: while doing research for the following chapter on negative ions, I came across an interesting piece of information. Fred Soyka—author of the seminal work entitled The Ion Effect—made a statement at a conference to the effect that, ions can be created by a natural phenomenon called "subterranean suspiration". Soyka said, "solar and lunar influences cause the water table to rise, forcing air out of the earth". He went on to explain that the air forced out of the earth is full of positive ions.

Since geopathic stress often occurs in areas where water flows underground, it is possible much of the negative influence of geopathic stress, can be attributed to the creation of high levels of positive ions. Therefore, increasing the negative ion flow in areas so affected may also alleviate some of the symptoms.

I have avoided going into the more esoteric components of geopathic stress, however (as with Feng Shui), it does also have metaphysical aspects. Therefore, if your home is uncomfortable because of unexplained phenomena—including anything that may be interpreted as "hauntings"—geopathic stress is something you will want to explore in more detail.

I will point out here electromagnetic pollution is the insult that adds to the injury of geopathic stress. We, in the West, have lost all memory of the principles of geopathic stress. We unthinkingly build anywhere, not considering the lay of the land. Thus, we have many homes and buildings located in high geopathic stress zones—adding the burden of electrosmog seriously worsens the health issues of those living in such homes.

CHAPTER SEVEN

NEGATIVE IONS AND EARTHING

IONS

An excess of positively charged ions can contribute to a variety of ailments, including constriction of the veins, depression, fatigue, and irritability. The opposite of positive ions are negative ions, which make your electrons spin in a clockwise direction, helping stabilize your cell membranes, and prevent oxidation (free radical damage). Thus, in this case, the "positive" has a negative effect, and the "negative" has a positive effect.

The existence of positive and negative ions was first identified by Dr. P.E.A. Lenard, who, in 1915, discovered that water, when atomized, separates the negative and positive charges. After an impact of a water droplet, the molecules discharged from the surface of the water carry a negative charge, and the remaining large drops of water carry the positive charge. This is why we find the highest natural sources of negative ions where water is being atomized.

Technically, a negative ion (anion) is an atom (or molecule) that has gained one, or more, extra negatively charged electrons. Negative ions are generated by sunlight, storms, rivers, ocean waves, waterfalls, and water evaporating after a rainfall. Even a shower will generate negative ions, which is the reason a shower is more invigo-rating than a bath.

A positive ion (cation), then, is an atom (or molecule) that has lost one, or more, electrons due to a high-energy impact. Natural forces that generate positive ions include, decaying radioactive ma-terials, radon gas, forest fires, lightning, and ultraviolet rays.

In the 1930s, a Russian scientist, A.L. Tchijevski, discovered he could reduce the growth of bacteria by subjecting it to negative ion exposure—a result of negative ions actually killing the bacteria. (Due to this research, many hospitals today use industrial-strength nega-tive ion machines to help maintain a germ-free environment.) By the time World War II broke out, German military planes had negative ion generators installed in them to prevent fatigue, and reduce the frequency of illness, in pilots.

POSITIVE IONS

There are places in the world where certain winds are considered almost evil. When these winds blow through an area, bad things happen—crime rates, hospital admissions, and suicides, all increase. As well, a wide range of symptoms show up in the general popula-tion, including breathing problems, depression, fatigue, irritability, inflammation, migraines, nausea, heart palpitations, sleep disorders, tremors, and vertigo.

These winds are known by different names in different coun-tries—Chinook in the Rockies, Santa Ana in Southern California, Sharav in Israel, and Simoon in Africa—but everywhere, results are the same: ill health. As these desert and sea winds tear through arid areas, the ensuing dust strips out negative ions, leaving about 33 times more positive ions—it is the presence of massive amounts of positive ions that causes these health problems.

Unnatural sources of positive ions include smog, cigarette smoke, indoor environments with poor circulation, vehicle interiors, any-thing plastic, electronic devices, and synthetic building materials,

K.W. PETERS

clothing, and furniture coverings. City living exposes us to unnaturally high levels of positive ions due to buildings, concrete, and pavement, all disrupting the electrical balance between the atmosphere and the earth. As a result, modern living has left us floating in a sea of positive ions.

Positive ions must balance themselves by collecting negative ions. Even though electronic devices put out massive amounts of positive ions, as long as there are plenty of negative ions around you (like fresh air, and plants), the positive ions will 'feed' on the natural negative ions, balancing their charge.

However, in the absence of negative ions, positive ions will go for the nearest thing that provides the missing component—they will steal negative ions from your body, causing mental, physical, and emotional imbalance. The widespread prevalence of electronics in modern life is creating a massive deficit in negative ions—another mechanism whereby they are proving to be detrimental to human well-being.

Positive ions increase levels of the inhibitory neurotransmitter, serotonin, in the body, and negative ions suppress serotonin levels. So, when the environment is depleted of negative ions, we experience the drowsiness and relaxation that comes with elevated serotonin levels. This may not be problematic at night, but is an issue during the day, when we need energy, alertness, and mental agility. What might be problematic at night is the tendency of positive ions to also cause inflammation, whereas negative ions can prevent this from occurring (or at least reduce the severity of it).

BENEFITS OF NEGATIVE IONS

Since the advent of negative ion machines, it has been possible to test the benefits of being exposed to high levels of these "good" ions. Of course, these "high" levels are really just close to what we would have been exposed to centuries ago, when we lived in nature—before the advent of modern cities.

Studies have found negative ions reduce anxiety and neurosis, improve appetite, and stimulate sexual behavior. And, they improve reaction time in drivers, reducing accident rates (you can buy small negative ion machines for cars, which plug into the cigarette lighter). In academic settings, negative ions improve learning capacity and mental functioning, reduce agitation in hyperactive children, and ameliorate teacher fatigue.

Negative ions, in medical settings, are used to alleviate hay fever symptoms, and migraines, and to reduce post-surgical pain. When burn victims are subjected to high levels of negative ions, they experience pain reduction, fewer infections, faster healing, and less scarring. And, some hospitals use the machines because of the demonstrated ability of negative ions to kill germs.

Many of the health benefits provided by negative ions are (theoretically) a result of them increasing our ability to absorb and utilize oxygen, thereby improving delivery of oxygen to the cells and tissues of the body.

CREATING NEGATIVE IONS

Since negative ions occur in nature, simply getting into nature frequently will allow you to breathe in these healing ions, reducing some of the effects of exposure to city living, and electrosmog. An especially good way to pick up negative ions is to go for a walk on the beach, through a forest, or anywhere after a rainstorm. Indoors, the most powerful negative ion generator you have is the shower, which, if you have a shower filter, can be used frequently to recharge yourself. If you do not have a shower filter, then the benefits of the negative ions must be weighed against the detriment of inhaling chlorine gas from city water.

It should be pointed out here that negative ions have to be inhaled on a regular basis to see the full benefits, and, since nature does not always provide enough to counteract modern living, a machine is more likely to be of value for those in poor health. Indeed, all of the research, referred to herein, was carried out, by necessity, with negative ion generating machines—so the subjects had continuous high-level exposure.

The other thing to be aware of is negative ions are best absorbed through the olfactory nerves. Thus, when attempting to absorb them, be sure to breathe in mostly through your nose, not through your mouth.

Try to keep a good flow of fresh air coming into your living, and work, spaces, in order to wash away positive ions, and keep levels of negative ions high. Plant leaves produce some negative ions, so the more plants you can have in your living and working spaces, the more protection you will have from electronically-produced positive ions.

Certain plants also remove toxins from the air. According to NASA research, some of the best ones are, bamboo palm, Chinese evergreen, English ivy, ficus (weeping fig), golden pothos, peace lily, philodendron, and spider plants. For best results, have at least one six-inch plant for every 100 square feet— though in this case, more is better.

Proponents of the Himalayan salt crystal lamps claim that they are natural negative ion producers, and that such devices flood the air with these ions when heated. In so doing, they redress any imbalance between positive and negative ions. These lamps do produce negative ions, as I have seen one analyzed with an ion detector, but the ions only radiated out for a couple of feet. Nonetheless, if you have a number of these salt lamps, and leave them on most of the time, the consistent production of negative ions should influence a room positively.

Pure beeswax is nontoxic, naturally aromatic, and, when burned as candles, emits beneficial negative ions, which help to purify the air. This does not hold true for petrochemical wax (used in most commercial candles), which is polluting in nature.

REDUCING POSITIVE IONS

It is a good idea to shut off electronic equipment, and fluorescent lights, when not in use. Otherwise, when left on, they will continue to deplete negative ions from the air, and increase the number of positive ions—leaving the environment ionically imbalanced. Unless you have a frequent flow of fresh air through it, a computer room will harbor about six times more positive than negative ions.

NEGATIVE ION MACHINES

Negative ions can be artificially generated by devices, which use an external electric power source to create large quantities of them. These negative ion generators went through a surge of popularity in North America, in the 1980s, and then faded into relative obscurity. However, they never fully went away because the benefits proved obvious to the users.

Now, it turns out, negative ions are part of our arsenal for fighting electrosmog, since electromagnetic pollution creates large amounts of positive ions. The irony of using an electronic device, to neutralize the detrimental effects of other electronic devices, is not lost on me. Fight fire with fire, they say. But, like with any electrical device, take care not to be too close to the negative ion generator when it is on, since it will still produce an electromagnetic field.

Most people in North America are not familiar with the negative ion concept, but in other parts of the world—especially Europe— such generators have been widely used for decades. In Germany, and Russia, negative ion generators are commonly found in factories, homes, hospitals, offices, restaurants, schools, spas, and vehicles. Whereas in the U.S., such machines are mostly found in submarines, and industrial settings, like auto spray paint booths, chemical spray factories, food processing plants, and grain storage bins.

You see, when there is a high enough concentration of negative ions in the air, they will attract positively-charged floating particles, in large numbers. This causes the particle to become too heavy to remain airborne. As a result, the particle will fall out of the air, and can then be collected by normal cleaning activities, such as vacuuming. This explains the prevalence of these devices in the aforementioned American industrial settings, where there are many airborne particles.

CHOOSING A MACHINE

There are many machines on the market designed to boost negative ions in the home, office, or vehicle. However, since this is a fairly unregulated area, with a lack of industry accepted and mandated standards, it is a case of "buyer beware".

For example, certain air purifiers will produce some negative ions, but those are produced inside the machine, and never actually enter the room. Many of the air purifiers that claim to produce negative ions are usually also ozone generators. Reading the fine print will reveal they only produce ozone, even though it will be implied they also create negative ions.

However, unlike negative ions, ozone is unstable, and easily destroyed by other pollutants in the air. Ozone never provides the benefits that true negative ions do. That being said, ozone is excellent at neutralizing airborne chemicals, strong odors, mold, and pollutants. So, these machines do have their place, as air cleaners.

However, be aware, excess ozone can be dangerous—so much so that you cannot safely remain in a room with an industrial-strength ozone machine operating. Nonetheless, these machines can be highly effective at removing serious mold, or mildew, build-up, in certain circumstances, and with the advice of a professional.

Therefore, before you buy any kind of negative ion generator, you will want to do your research. Be sure to read any informative material provided, from package details, to a manual, if available. Find forums, and/or customer reviews, on a given product, to ensure it has satisfied customers.

I did some research (given the debatable quality of some negative ion machines), and can confidently recommend the very affordable Comtech product (price range: $150 to $200). (www.comtech-pcs. com)

A more expensive product—the kind used in hospital—is the ELANRA Therapeutic Ionizer, produced by Bionic Products in Australia (since 1967). Trademarked, and patented internationally, ELANRA Ionizers claim to be the number one medical ionizer in the world. The cost ranges from $800 to $1,000, for home units. (www. negativeions.com)

The ELANRA Ionizer defines its quality by the size of the negative ions it produces. While medium to large negative ions will clean the air, only the small ions are biologically active—which means these small ions can be breathed in, and will enter the bloodstream by way of the lungs.

As an interesting side note, literature on the ELANRA Ionizer claims that within one minute of exposure to the unit, the "Schumann Resonance" was detected in the brain waves of humans. This frequency (the one the earth resonates at), is something missing from modern life, as we are separated from the earth by concrete, pavement, houses, and shoes.

For the full story on negative ions, I recommend reading The Ion Effect, by Fred Soyka.

EARTHING: ONE SOLUTION TO ELECTROPOLLUTION

There is another natural way of getting more negative ions into your life, which is known as "Earthing".

When we are out of the city, not only do we absorb negative ions, but we are also more connected to the Earth's own electromagnetic frequency—the aforementioned Schumann Resonance—at exactly 7.83 hertz. Not surprisingly, this is the same frequency at which our brains, and bodies, function optimally, and it is a big part of why it feels so good to be in nature.

When I first started studying the Japanese health system known as Macrobiotics, I was curious about one of their recommendations for health and vitality. The suggestion was to walk barefoot in dewy grass, first thing in the morning, for at least 10 minutes. I never really practiced that suggestion much, but I always remembered it, and recently I have found out why it was such a valid concept.

Humans have walked barefoot (or in footwear made of natural materials), and slept on the ground, throughout the majority of our existence. This kept us directly in contact with the Earth's magnetic field. But, now that we no longer sleep on the ground, and we wear insulating rubber, or plastic-soled, shoes, we have been disconnected from the Earth's energy field.

The concept of "Earthing" raises the possibility that this disconnection may be directly linked to chronic pain, extreme fatigue, and the poor sleeping patterns prevalent in modern life. It is part of the natural order for our bodies to be in contact with the Earth, and in order to function properly we need to maintain this connection as much as possible.

THE BODY ELECTRIC

As discussed in the chapter on electrosmog, every living creature is a collection of electrical circuits, with all of our cells transmitting and receiving energy, by way of essential biochemical reactions. Electric fields regulate the movement of nutrients and water into the cells, and all of our actions, behaviors, and movements, are dependent on these electrical exchanges.

The brain, heart, muscles, immune, and nervous systems, all operate based on bioelectrical subsystems within our bodies. All external physical electrical systems used in the world have to be *grounded* (stabilized by the Earth's electrical energy) in order to work properly. In a similar manner, when a body is connected to the Earth, it receives an electric signal that normalizes, and stabilizes, its bioelectrical systems.

Currently, the widespread electromagnetic pollution we are subject to is wreaking havoc on our body's normal bioelectrical field. Though this constant invisible assault is linked to many ailments, the Earthing concept suggests there is a partial solution to electrosmog, which will help us feel better, sleep better, and have more balanced energy levels.

The simple approach to Earthing is to sit, or walk barefoot, on the earth, whenever possible, in order to reestablish that connection to the Earth's magnetic field. The more modern (and convenient) approach is to sleep, work, and/or relax, indoors, while being in contact with conductive sheets, or mats, that are grounded to the earth. These grounding devices both discharge the unhealthy voltage we carry in our bodies from electromagnetic pollution, and transfer the healing energy of the Earth into our bodies.

REDISCOVERING EARTHING

It turns out Macrobiotics was not the only traditional healing system aware of the concept of Earthing. Other cultures have also observed the benefits of grounding to the Earth. They identified this Earth energy in different ways, including "Earth Chi", found in Traditional Chinese Medicine, and "Prana", found in the East Indian medical tradition of Ayurveda. In the West, this concept has been brought to the fore mostly due to the pioneering work of Clint Ober, and his book on the subject: "Earthing: The Most Important Health Discovery Ever?" (Clinton Ober, Stephen T. Sinatra, M.D. and Martin Zucker).

Clint Ober, an early member of the cable TV industry, became seriously ill at the age of 49. After his recovery, he decided to reinvent himself. He rid himself of most of his possessions, and traveled around America in a recreational vehicle for four years, looking for a higher purpose in life. One day, while simply observing a passing parade of people, he noticed almost everyone was wearing synthetic-soled shoes. Ober began to wonder if synthetic footwear—having almost exclusively replaced leather—could be having a negative effect on health, because, in effect, it insulated everybody from the electrical surface charge of the Earth.

Ober's work in cable TV reminded him that, before cable, TV images often were contaminated with flecks of static, or lines across the screen, due to electromagnetic interference. Now cable systems are grounded, and shielded, in order to prevent outside signals, and fields, from interfering with the transmission of TV signals being carried through the cable. This cable shield is connected to the Earth via a grounding rod, as are the electrical systems found in homes, buildings, and industry—in order to provide electrical stability.

Ober suspected this energy field might also protect the human body from the dangers of electromagnetic pollution. Since he already knew the body conducts electricity, he decided to try a simple experiment on himself. He attached an alligator clip to a copper grid, connected a wire to it, ran the wire out the window, and attached it to a ground rod, set in the earth outside. Then he measured the voltage on his body with a voltage meter, and found that, when he was grounded, the electro-magnetic fields previously registering on his body had disappeared, leaving his body with the same voltage level as the surface of the Earth.

Ober slept on the grounding grid, and, by morning, he found he had fallen asleep, and slept soundly, for the first time in a long time—without the painkillers he usually needed to sleep through the night. He repeated the experiment every night for a week with the same positive results, also noticing a significant decrease in his pain levels. Next, he started trying the system out on friends and acquaintances, who also found their sleep patterns improved, and their pain levels dropped.

He went on to organize studies with scientists that validated his initial observations of improved sleep, and reduced pain levels. As he worked, over the next decade, to validate his theories, he also further developed and refined his indoor Earthing system, both for use in the studies, and to make the system available to people who needed it.

The Earthing products Ober developed are available at www. earthing.com, and include sheets, blankets, pads for the feet (to be used while on the computer). They also offer patches, which can be directly attached to the body, for targeting specific areas that are inflamed. These products have two grounding options: one that goes to a metal rod, which is put into the ground, outside, and one that goes to the grounding port in a regular electrical outlet.

INFLAMMATION

Many modern diseases share the same root cause: chronic inflammation. When inflammation continues after the healing process— sometimes for years—tissue damage occurs, and the body exhausts its energy levels, and immune functions, trying to cope with it.

Inflammation is due, in part, to free radicals, which are positively-charged molecules. Since the Earth is putting off negatively-charged electrons, which, when they are absorbed into our body, neutralize such free radicals, Earthing can be used to reduce inflammation. This theory is supported both by research, and by feedback from countless people who have used the Earthing technique, and/ or the grounding products, to reduce inflammation in their bodies.

Ever since the use of rubber, and plastic-soled, shoes became widespread, replacing the old-fashioned leather soles (which conduct the Earth's energy), most people spend very little time in actual contact with the Earth. Add to that the non-conductive flooring of our buildings, and the time we spend in vehicles, and the result is most of us seldom touch the Earth—with the exception of tropical vacations, or the occasional trip to the beach in summer.

Being insulated from the natural magnetic frequency of the Earth leaves us "electron deficient", which in turn leads to an excess of free radicals in the body, resulting in chronic inflammation. Diseases linked to inflammation include allergies, Alzheimer's, arthritis, asthma, cancer, Crohn's, colitis, diabetes, eczema, heart disease, fibromyalgia, lupus, MS, and psoriasis.

On the other hand, when we have an adequate supply of negatively-charged electrons in our bodies, an antioxidant effect occurs that keeps our immune system functioning, and protects our body from inflammation, and free radical damage. Keep in mind, free radical damage is linked to premature aging, as well as to most serious diseases.

BENEFITS OF EARTHING

In a blog about Earthing, psychiatrist Tracy Latz M.D. talked about recommending this technique to her patients, as part of a total program, mentioning how it has improved health in many cases. She writes, "Patients who do follow my recommendation to 'Earth', and there have been dozens of them, tend to have good responses. They are individuals with a wide variety of emotional, mental, and physical problems, and often combinations of problems. They often tell me afterward they feel much better". She finds the first thing they notice is better sleep patterns.

By improving sleep, Earthing helps normalize serotonin levels, and lower cortisol levels. This gives those with anxiety issues an "improved sense of safety". When cortisol levels are too high, we easily fall into anxiety as a response to any stressful situation, and/or respond with irritability, or anger. When cortisol levels return to normal, we find it easier to be calm and peaceful, and to respond to stressful situations with a balanced attitude.

When our serotonin levels are balanced, we are less likely to be depressed, and more likely to avoid obsessive and repetitive, negative thoughts. Our energy level improves, as does our tolerance to stressful situations, and pain. Indeed, Dr. Latz has also found that patients with chronic pain have benefitted from Earthing, as well as those suffering from other inflammatory conditions (including gluten intolerance, and IBS).

While not a total cure for these conditions, the practice of Earthing reduces symptoms, making such ailments at least easier to manage. She also recommends Earthing to those with autoimmune conditions, fibromyalgia, chronic fatigue syndrome, and even to athletes for recovery from injuries, and muscle inflammation.

According to the website, www.earthingcanada.ca (Canadian distributor for these products), research and testimonials indicate Earthing can offer the following benefits:

- Better sleep patterns, including falling asleep more easily, not waking up frequently during the night, and feeling more rested in the morning.

- Reduction or elimination of muscle stiffness, and back and joint pain.

- A more balanced mood with fewer episodes of anxiety, depression, and irritability, and improved energy throughout the day.

- Reduced gastrointestinal symptoms.

- Reduction in symptoms of menopause and PMS.

- Elimination of jet lag.

THE SCIENCE

There have been some actual scientific studies done on Earthing, a number of which can be found at the following web address: www.hindawi.com/journals/jeph/2012/291541.

One double-blind study examined sleep and chronic pain in 60 subjects who had serious sleep disorders, along with consistent joint and muscle pain. The patients who received proper grounding showed relief from these health problems, while the majority of the control group did not. The Earthing benefits also ranged well beyond just sleep and pain control; other conditions that also showed improvement, included relief from asthmatic and respiratory conditions, hypertension, rheumatoid arthritis, PMS, and sleep apnea.

The conclusion of this study was as follows, "Emerging evidence shows that contact with the Earth—whether being outside barefoot or indoors connected to grounded conductive systems—may be a simple, natural, and yet profoundly effective environmental strategy against chronic stress, ANS dysfunction, inflammation, pain, poor sleep, disturbed HRV, hypercoagulable blood, and many common health disorders, including cardiovascular disease. The research done to date supports the concept that grounding or Earthing the human body may be an essential element in the health equation along with sunshine, clean air and water, nutritious food, and physical activity".(1)

Seeking to discover if Earthing could be helpful in preventing heart disease, another study looked at the effects of 2 hours of grounding on the electrical charge on red blood cells (RBCs). The conclusion was as follows, "Grounding increases the surface charge on RBCs and thereby reduces blood viscosity and clumping. Grounding appears to be one of the simplest and yet most profound interventions for helping reduce cardiovascular risk and cardiovascular events". (2)

DO IT YOURSELF

I have talked with people who have experienced the benefits of natural Earthing on pain levels, and inflammation, and I have some personal experience as well. So I have no doubt this is a valid theory. To try it yourself, simply go outside and stand, walk, sit, and/or lay, on the grass, ground, or beach, for at least half an hour, and see what kind of difference it makes on your pain or stress levels.

Bare flesh on the ground is best, but ions will also transfer through natural fabric. The feet will conduct better through socks, than sitting on the ground with pants on, because the feet tend to be moist, due to perspiration—and moisture allows for an easier transfer of electrons. Having your hands in direct contact with the earth is also highly effective.

Because the body is mostly water and minerals, it is a good conductor of electricity. And, in the absence of barriers, free electrons on the surface of the Earth transfer easily to the human body—as long as there is direct contact. When there is moisture present, the transfer is even easier, and faster, so having contact with damp grass, soil, or sand, is more effective than a totally dry surface. Of course swimming, or putting your feet into the ocean, lake, or a river, is also an excellent way to practice Earthing.

Leather-soled shoes are not quite as good as bare feet for grounding, but are certainly better than standard rubber, or plastic soles. Even though leather itself is not conductive, perspiration from the foot allows energy from the Earth to conduct up through it, and into the body. Moisture from walking on damp ground, or sidewalks, can also help electrons permeate up through leather-soled shoes. However, a very thick leather sole may not allow sufficient moisture through, so a thinner soled moccasin is the best type of conductive footwear for walking on the earth.

Wood, asphalt, plastic, rubber, and vinyl, are not conductive surfaces, so you will not receive any Earthing benefits from time spent on them. However, concrete is a conductive material (if it is not painted or sealed), since it is made of water and minerals, and it rests on the Earth, and holds moisture. Thus, we can pick up ions when on concrete, as long as there are not any non-conductive materials between us and the concrete.

DOES IT WORK FOR EVERYONE?

Some individuals report feeling a strange, buzzing energy, when they start Earthing, especially those who are hypersensitive. Makers of grounding devices suggest this is often part of a temporary detoxification process, and usually this feeling will dissipate as their body becomes adjusted to the Earth's energy field.

If you should have this response, and it is too uncomfortable, start by only spending 5 to 15 minutes grounded (whether outside, or with the devices). Then gradually increasing your exposure until you become more comfortable with it. Not everyone needs the same amount of exposure to receive benefits, so even if you cannot work up to regular exposure, or cannot use it during sleep, you may still reap the benefits of Earthing. It is suggested that people who are highly electro-sensitive should use the grounding rod (planted directly into the earth) version of Earthing devices, rather than the grounding port, which is plugged into a 3-pronged electrical outlet.

THE DOWNSIDE OF EARTHING

Now, let's look briefly at the counter argument (these days, there is always a counter argument). There are EMF experts who disagree with the use of Earthing sheets and mats, and who believe that, if we do use them, at the very least they must be grounded into the earth, not into the wall socket. Their theory is, when we plug the Earthing mat, or sheet, into the electrical socket, we are connecting to the ground of our houses' electrical wiring, and thus tapping into all the different frequencies running through that wiring—which includes the fluctuating dirty electricity frequencies.

Critics of Earthing products believe these bad frequencies, coursing through electrical wiring, will run back up through the grounding wire, adding more electromagnetic pollution to our bodies. They maintain this is the reason hypersensitive people often have a negative response to Earthing products that are plugged into the wall—often experiencing agitation, fatigue, restless legs, and/or poor sleep patterns.

The marketing of Earthing products includes videos illustrating that a voltage meter will show a reduction of the body's electrical fields, when people touch a grounding mat, or sheet. However, this decline does not necessarily mean one is protected—it can just indicate that the field is reduced, because your body is connected to the ground. According to this theory, you are now just part of the path the electromagnetic frequencies take on their way to the Earth.

Some also believe that the grounding sheets, because they are made with conductive metal threads, can work as an antenna for radio frequency radiation, pulling more out of the air—again, increasing our total load of electrosmog.

From that perspective, it appears Earthing products should ideally be connected to the type of ground that is placed in the earth outside (clearly something that only works if you live in a house, or an apartment at ground level). Other than that, you want to be sure your home has been tested for electromagnetic pollution, and dirty electricity, and that everything which can be done to lower it to a manageable level, has been done. In other words, you want a very electrosmog-free home before you ground out an Earthing product into the electric socket, or it may be counterproductive.

One other potential problem is, not all outside ground is free of electric charge. If the area has been disturbed by construction, has metal pipes running nearby, or is near a power plant, the ground there can be polluted by electric charges—resulting in compromised grounding.

Fortunately, if you buy an Earthing product from the website, they do offer a money-back guarantee, so if you find it does not work for you, you have recourse. The best approach is to simply try it, and see if it makes you feel better, or not.

My electrosensitive friend, while living close to banks of cell phone towers, still found using the Earthing sheet made a big difference in helping her sleep. Given this, and other feedback, I personally believe Earthing products are worth testing out, and can offer many benefits, to most people. I certainly have never experienced any negative effects from my Earthing sheet.

Even though we may derive some protection, and health benefits, from grounding and Earthing, it would be foolish to think that this is sufficient to combat all electro-magnetic pollution. For some people, Earthing solutions may be all they need to deal with mild electrosmog exposure, while others, with greater exposure, and/or

K.W. PETERS

hypersensitivity, may find it offers some relief, but may need to incorporate other measures as well. Either way, the safest way to practice Earthing is certainly to get regular physical contact with the Earth.

Endnotes

1. Journal of Environmental and Public Health; Volume 2012 (2012), Article ID 291541, Review Article Earthing: Health Implications of Reconnecting the Human Body to the Earth's Surface Electrons; Gaétan Chevalier, et al.
2. The Journal of Alternative and Complementary Medicine; 2012, "Earthing (Grounding) the Human Body Reduces Blood Viscosity—a Major Factor in Cardiovascular Disease." Gaetan Chevalier, et al.

CHAPTER EIGHT

CONCLUSION

Please do not think this is a comprehensive account of all the invisible dangers we face in the modern world, or that I have covered all of the solutions. As this book grew, over the course of the last 6 years, I found such a continuous influx of new material it seemed like there was more and more information I needed to include—information revealing both new dangers, and new solutions.

I eventually realized that new information on these subjects would be endless, and it was time to stop accumulating data, and share the basic material I had gathered. So, while I believe I have provided enough data to be of service, it is advisable for readers to continue to update themselves on information related to the subjects covered herein. Related information can be found in my blogs, and newsletters, at www.nutristart.com, and from alternative websites, such as www.greenmedinfo.com.

As I wrote, and rewrote, this book, over the years, revisiting the material and adding new discoveries, it started to feel like I was living in a science fiction movie. A movie akin to "The Matrix"—wherein most people live in a highly unnatural, constructed-reality, of which they are completely unaware.

That being said, I have not even included the extreme viewpoints of those inclined to conspiratorial beliefs. They ask why the energy output, and quantity, of cell phone antennas, is far greater than the communication requirements of smartphones.

Check out the number of cell phone antennas in your city (look up; they are clustered atop businesses, and apartment buildings), and ask yourself if it seems there are far more than could possibly be necessary for simple communication needs, and internet access.

To get a real sense of this, check out the website www.ertyu.org, and look for the "Canadian Cellular Towers Map". This is a map of all the cell phone towers in Canada (I am sure such maps are available online for other countries as well), and it is shocking to see it visually represented. What is even more shocking is zooming in on an area, and clicking on one of the pins that indicate a cell tower location (they are color-coded, based on which cellular provider owns them). Now click on the provider's name that comes up, and you will find that the pin represents anywhere from one to 18 (the highest count I found) cellular antennas, at that particular location.

I used this map to examine an apartment building I knew had a number of cell phone antennas on it (a concern to the tenants living there). This apartment building is government-subsidized housing for the most fragile among us (seniors, and those with disabilities). On top of this building were 18 antennas belonging to one cellular provider and 18 antennas belonging to another.

Installing these antennas provides the government with a few extra dollars, but no one in that bureaucracy is willing to listen to the concerns of the tenants. Yet, those tenants I spoke with discussed the increased frequency of deaths, and hospitalizations, occurring among the long-term residents, since the installation of the antennas. These tenants also voiced concerns that their personal health was being negatively affected, but, of course, the majority of them do not have the resources to move.

As if our current electrosmog overload were not bad enough, there is a new wave of wireless technology on the horizon, which could be in place as early as 2021. In March 2016, the U.S. passed the

"Mobile Now Act", paving the way for plans to expand 5G mobile broadband throughout the country.

In Canada, newspapers reported that, "Bell, Rogers and Telus are all participating in a global effort to develop operating standards for fifth generation (5G) wireless networks, with Bell Canada set to begin testing of the emerging architecture".

While 5G speed will provide advantages for technology and communications, there are many concerned experts predicting widespread implementation of 5G technology will pose even greater health risks than current wireless technology already does.

The Federal Communications Commission in the U.S. is pushing to streamline approval of 5G cell towers, authorizing these experimental high frequencies to be implemented without proper safety testing. These untested frequencies, in the range of 28 to 100 gigahertz, or more, could soon be everywhere, since they require a massive deployment of small cell towers.

To take the science fiction analogy further, there are those who theorize that even the current situation (of countless, overpowered cell phone antenna arrays) can be used in conjunction with extremely low frequency (ELF) systems (like the HAARP project), for weather manipulation, and widespread mind control of the general population. (For an overview of the aforementioned conspiratorial ideas about weather manipulation, and mind control, check out: www.earthpulse.com.)

So, I stayed within the range of acknowledged (if often ignored, or denied) science, and still it feels like a science fiction movie. Especially when my electrosensitive friend demonstrates her hypersensitivity to these fields, I see how damaging they are to her life, and I speak with others in the same (sinking) boat.

Unlike the Iroquois idea of "Seven generation stewardship"—a concept that encourages the present generation of humans to live and work for the benefit of the seventh generation into the future—our leaders, both in business and politics, pay no attention to the long-term ramifications of their decisions.

Currently, business decisions are based on attaining the highest level of immediate profit possible, especially when shareholders must be answered to. Political decisions are motivated by getting elected four years hence; few politicians are willing to sacrifice in the short-term for long-term benefit—though all too many are willing to sell out the future for present gains.

However, it is not my goal to spread fear, but rather to empower the average person; after all, forewarned is forearmed. What I have attempted to do is to provide strategies you can use to protect the health of both you and your loved ones, in the face of these invisible assaults. It is my hope you will then share this knowledge with other open-minded people.

In closing, I would like to point out that, for those who are seriously ill, there are factors other than diet, and supplements, which must be considered. Our weaknesses (often constitutional) determine where illness strikes. Inflammation, for example—whether due to poor diet, nutritional deficiencies, and/or electromagnetic pollution—may cause arthritis in one person, diabetes in another, or cancer in others, depending on their genetic predisposition.

We are all unique, and maintaining good health, or reversing illness, must include addressing the needs of body, mind, and spirit, in whatever way resonates most strongly with you. Thus, bodywork—yoga, Tai Chi, massage therapy, etc.—is an important component of healing physical ailments, just as exercise is a necessary component of maintaining general health.

Emotional work—Jungian therapy, Emotional Freedom Technique, Neuro-linguistic programming, and so on—is a necessary component for serious ailments that involve unhealthy mental states, or nervous disorders, just as having a healthy social network of friends and family is required for general well-being.

Finally, for life-threatening, or seemingly unsolvable, illnesses, we must incorporate energy work—Reiki, Auric balancing, Qi Gong, etc—in order to address the underlying roots of illness, just as for day-to-day well being we need to fulfill our spiritual needs. We need not be religious in order to serve our spiritual component—in fact, in the case of fundamentalist religious beliefs, I believe religion to be counter to Spirit. However, we unquestionably have this built-in facility, and, whether it is God-given, or a by-product of evolution, it must be acknowledged and fulfilled, for us to be truly healthy and happy people.

Such subjects are beyond the scope of this book, but I suggest that you do not think of them as foolish, or unnecessary. Remember that Newtonian physics, which implies we all just exist in a clockwork universe, has proven to be insufficient to explain the universe. While quantum physics, which implies that we are co-creators of our reality, has brought us one large step closer to understanding life, and its inherent meaning.

For last words, I will leave you with a quotation that often provide solace for those who feel they don't fit into society, and who feel confused about holding views contrary to the majority:

> *It is no measure of health to be well-adjusted to a profoundly sick society.*
>
> *J. Krishnamurti*